Clinical Management
of the Perimenopause

Clinical Management
of the Perimenopause

Edited by

Shawky ZA Badawy

Professor and Chairman, Department of Obstetrics
and Gynecology,
Professor, Department of Pathology,
Director, Division of Reproductive Endocrinology
and Infertility,
State University of New York Health Science Center
at Syracuse, Syracuse, New York, USA

ARNOLD

A member of the Hodder Headline Group
LONDON • SYDNEY • AUCKLAND
Co-published in the United States of America by
Oxford University Press Inc., New York

First published in Great Britain in 1999 by
Arnold, a member of the Hodder Headline Group,
338 Euston Road, London NW1 3BH

http://www.arnoldpublishers.com

Co-published in the United States of America by
Oxford University Press Inc.,
198 Madison Avenue, New York, NY10016
Oxford is a registered trademark of Oxford University Press

Whilst the advice and information in this book are believed to be true and
accurate at the date of going to press, neither the authors nor the publisher
can accept any legal responsibility or liability for any errors or omissions
that may be made. In particular (but without limiting the generality of the
preceding disclaimer) every effort has been made to check drug dosages;
however, it is still possible that errors have been missed. Furthermore,
dosage schedules are constantly being revised and new side-effects
recognized. For these reasons the reader is strongly urged to consult the
drug companies' printed instructions before administering any of the drugs
recommended in this book.

British Library Cataloguing in Publication Data
A catalogue record for this book is available from the British Library

Library of Congress Cataloging-in-Publication Data
A catalog record for this book is available from the Library of Congress

ISBN 0 340 74150 3

1 2 3 4 5 6 7 8 9 10

Commissioning Editor: Jo Koster
Production Editor: Rada Radojicic
Production Controller: Priya Gohil

Typeset in Minion by J&L Composition Ltd, Filey, North Yorkshire
Printed in Great Britain by St Edmundsbury Press, Suffolk
Bound in Great Britain by MPG Books, Bodmin, Cornwall

What do you think about this book? Or any other Arnold title?
Please send your comments to feedback.arnold@hodder.co.uk

Contents

Contributors

EDITOR

Shawky ZA Badawy MD
Professor and Chairman, Department of Obstetrics and Gynecology, Professor, Department of Pathology, Director, Division of Reproductive Endocrinology and Infertility, State University of New York Health Science Center at Syracuse, Syracuse, New York, USA

CONTRIBUTORS

Raja W Abdul-Karim MD
Professor of Obstetrics and Gynecology, State University of New York Health Science Center at Syracuse, Syracuse, New York, USA

Fatma A Aleem MD, PhD
Professor of Obstetrics and Gynecology, State University of New York, Director of Reproductive Endocrinology and Menopause, Brookdale University Hospital and Medical Center, Brooklyn, New York, USA

Michal Artal MD
Assistant Professor, Department of Psychiatry, Saint Louis University Health Sciences Center, USA

Samuel S Badalian MD, PhD
Department of Obstetrics and Gynecology, State University of New York Health Science Center at Syracuse, Syracuse, New York, USA

Philip J Buckenmeyer PhD
Department Coordinator, Assistant Professor and Director, Human Performance Laboratory, Department of Physical and Health Education, The University of Akron, Akron, Ohio, USA

Mary J Cunningham MD
Associate Professor, Director, Division of Gynecologic Oncology, Department of Obstetrics and Gynecology, State University of New York Health Science Center at Syracuse, Syracuse, New York, USA

Giovanni Elia MD
Assistant Professor, Department of Obstetrics and Gynecology, Director, Division of Urogynecology, State University of New York Health Science Center at Syracuse, Syracuse, New York, USA

Christine M Finck MD
Surgical Resident, Department of Surgery, State University of New York Health Science Center at Syracuse, Syracuse, New York, USA

Loren B Frankel MD
Resident Physician, Department of Obstetrics and Gynecology, State University of New York Health Science Center at Syracuse, Syracuse, New York, USA

Richard J Ham MD
State University of New York Distinguished Chair in Geriatric Medicine, Program in Geriatrics, Professor of Family Medicine, Department of Medicine, State University of New York Health Science Center at Syracuse, Syracuse, New York, USA

Gregory R Harper MD, PhD
Director, John and Dorothy Morgan Cancer Center, Professor of Clinical Medicine, Penn State University College of Medicine, John and Dorothy Morgan Cancer Center, Allentown, PA, USA

Alessandro Laviano MD
Department of Clinical Medicine, University of Rome 'La Sapienza', Rome, Italy

Shylaja Maini MD
Department of Surgery, State University of New York Health Science Center at Syracuse, Syracuse, New York, USA

Zahi N Makhuli MD
Associate Professor of Urology, State University of New York Health Science Center at Syracuse, Syracuse, New York, USA

Michael M Meguid MD, PhD, FACS
Comprehensive Breast Care Program, Department of Surgery, State University of New York Health Science Center at Syracuse, Syracuse, New York, USA

Robert EL Nesbitt Jr, MD
Professor Emeritus, Department of Obstetrics and Gynecology, State University of New York Health Science Center at Syracuse, Syracuse, New York, USA

Patricia J Numann MD
Professor of Surgery, Department of Surgery, State University of New York Health Science Center at Syracuse, Syracuse, New York, USA

Manvinder Singh MD
Assistant Professor, Department of Obstetrics and Gynecology, Division of Reproductive Endocrinology and Infertility, State University of New York Health Science Center at Syracuse, Syracuse, New York, USA

Preface

Victor Hugo, in his widely-quoted preface to a published work of Cromwell, downgraded his own contribution by pointing out that one seldom inspects the cellar of a house after visiting its salons nor examines the roots of a tree after eating the fruit. Without question, the organization, substance, and style of this book will speak eloquently and authoritatively on its own behalf. However, as one whose professional life in medicine has spanned more than half of this century, I have found compelling the opportunity to provide a portal to the important subject matter given thorough treatment in this compendium.

As we stand upon the threshold of a new millennium at a pivotal time that is a bridge between two centuries, our attention is drawn to the turbulent undercurrents of unprecedented technology, telecommunications, and social change. More than ever before, the medical philosophy of Virchow rings true. In 1849 he wrote, 'Should medicine ever fulfil its great ends, it must enter into the larger political and social life of our time.' In his further discourse, Virchow charged medicine with the obligation to 'indicate the barriers which obstruct the normal completion of the lifestyle and remove them.' This call for innovative approaches to new kinds of patients and situations pertains directly to today's woman, regardless of age, who expects to pursue a varied lifestyle within a society open to opportunities that go beyond the activities of home and family. Perimenopausal women, who are enjoying an extended life span, improved health, and more time and viable options for self-expression, are now emphasizing behavioral modifications that focus on the quality of their life.

Thus, medicine in general must move beyond the insular world of biotechnological applications and the hallowed halls of academia to redefine its value system and mission to become a profession of privileged servants who recognize that they are entrusted with sacred duty. Senator William H. Frist, MD put it best. 'The ideal of physician as leader is greater than any one of us, but it begins with each of us.' We must rise above the recognition of our 'monuments of unageing intellect,' as the Irish poet W.B. Yeats put it, to give full expression to our latent capacities for human understanding and pay tribute to services based on compassionate relationships. The new millennium challenges us to search for more coherence in the world and to focus greater attention on the whole and fullness of humanity beginning with just one person in want of care. At the same time, our record of service must verify that we have 'shared as little as any in the defects of the period.' (Robert Louis Stevenson).

It is well known that all the literary and performing arts, whether they be novels, poetry, drama, or any form that embodies 'creative and imaginative literature,' as Swinburne refers to it, will provide the best social commentary concerning the status and relevance of health care in that period. Dissertations about today's active women will also provoke postscripts to medicine about its accommodations to the new lifestyles that evolved during the course of their perimenopausal years. Standards set now by modern-day physicians can become the bellwether for future health professionals who must be responsive to the crosscurrents of social dynamics that will reshape the coming new age.

Dr Badawy, together with distinguished academic colleagues who represent all relevant disciplines pertaining to the health care of perimenopausal women, has compiled the first multifaceted, comprehensive work on the subject. The clinical and basic material is covered in sufficient depth and scope to prepare students and clinicians alike for the demanding medical responsibilities that will be required of twenty-first-century physicians. These authors, who have given substance and practical reality to the clear vision of Dr Badawy at a portentous moment in human history, deserve high praise for their cooperative efforts and individual contributions.

Robert E.L. Nesbitt Jr, MD
Professor Emeritus
Department of Obstetrics and Gynecology
State University of New York
Health Science Center at Syracuse

1

The pathophysiology of perimenopause

SHAWKY ZA BADAWY AND LOREN B FRANKEL

INTRODUCTION

The life span of women in the United States has changed significantly during the twentieth century. In the year 1900, the life expectancy of women was 47 to 50 years; by the year 1990, the life span of women was 75 to 80 years. Despite the increased life expectancy, the age of onset of menopause has not changed and has remained at between 50 and 52 years. Women will spend about 30 or more years of their lives in the stages known as menopause and postmenopause.[1-3]

There have also been changes in the social status of women during the century. Earlier in the century women used to marry at a young age and have large families. More recently, women have delayed their childbearing to a relatively older age while limiting the number of children per family. More women are seeking careers and looking to build a stable future for themselves before starting their families.[4]

Primary care physicians, therefore, should look at the whole spectrum of women's lives and try to identify each stage with its specific medical needs. The reproductive years of women have been well reviewed with regard to contraception, fertility studies, protection against sexually transmitted diseases and exercise-related changes. Furthermore, the menopause and postmenopause are also well addressed in the medical literature with regard to hormone replacement therapy and its advantages and disadvantages. However, menopause is not an abrupt phenomenon. There is a stage in women's lives which is considered to be transitional between the end of the reproductive years and the beginning of the menopause. This stage of life may vary between a few years or up to ten years, and comprises various changes which need to be addressed, diagnosed and treated adequately in order to improve quality of life and lead to a smooth entry into the menopausal years.

There has been an increase in the number of perimenopausal women. It is well known that the number of these women who will present to primary care physician offices will also be increased in the next century. It has also been found that 10% of women do not experience that stage of perimenopause, but enter directly into the menopausal stage. The remainder of the women will experience problems related to perimenopause, including vasomotor symptoms, irregular uterine bleeding, disturbances in sleep, psychological problems and bone-related problems.

ENDOCRINOLOGY

The endocrine changes that occur in the perimenopausal years are related to the aging of the hypothalamic–pituitary ovarian axis. It is estimated that the ovary of the newborn female contains about one million to two million oocytes. By the age of onset of puberty, the ovary will contain about 300,000 to 400,000 oocytes. Most of these oocytes are used during the reproductive years in the process of ovulation. By the age of 40, about a few thousand of these oocytes remain. Due to this, the process of ovulation occurs irregularly as compared to the reproductive years. This constitutes the basis of the cycle irregularity and the prevalence of abnormal uterine bleeding in this stage of a woman's life.

During the reproductive years, there is a continuous interaction between the ovarian hormones and the gonadotropins. The levels of both follicle-stimulating hormone (FSH) and luteinizing hormone (LH) remain at a normal range within the cycle and rise only around ovulation in what are known as FSH and LH peaks. Studies have shown that FSH and LH levels gradually increase, starting at the age of 29 to 30. By the age of 40 years, both FSH and LH levels are significantly higher compared to the years before.[5,6] This rise may be related to the gradual decline in the number of oocytes and also to the reduction in the levels of inhibin, which is produced by the granulosa cells. In addition, studies have documented the existence of low gonadotropin receptor levels in the perimenopausal ovaries.[7]

The measurement of baseline FSH levels with the onset of menses is usually helpful to predict the capability of the ovary to respond to gonadotropin stimulation in the infertile population during perimenopause. Elevated FSH in the perimenopause suggests that the ovarian reserve is on the decline and that the response to ovarian stimulation will be less favorable than in patients below the age of 40. As a result of changes in gonadotropin levels, serum estradiol levels in this age group tend to fluctuate between a normal range and a subnormal range. This is related to reduction in the total number of follicles within the aging ovary and a qualitative reduction in the ability of the granulosa cells to secrete hormones.[8]

As a result of decreased steroidogenesis by the ovarian follicles, there will be an increase in gonadotropin-releasing hormone (GNRH) pulsatility. This will lead to an increase in FSH and LH levels. This confirms the age-related exaggerated pituitary response to GNRH stimulation in women over the age of 30 and in the perimeno-pausal years. The subtle gonadotropin elevations in the perimenopausal years signal a declining ovarian reserve. This will affect both fertility and uterine bleeding in this age group.

Oligo-ovulatory cycles are common during perimenopausal years. The lack of ovulation leads to marked decline in progesterone levels in some cycles, causing irregular uterine bleeding, marked endometrial proliferation and hyperplasia.

CLINICAL MANIFESTATIONS

Dysfunctional uterine bleeding

This is defined as abnormal uterine bleeding not related to pregnancy or its complications and not associated with any organic disease in the genital tract. The majority of these cases are due to anovulatory cycles. Very rarely they occur in ovulatory cycles in which the progesterone secretion by the corpus luteum is insufficient and uterine bleeding occurs.[9]

The main pathology in anovulatory cycles is the exposure of the endometrium to unopposed estrogen. This will lead to continued endometrial proliferation with subsequent endometrial hyperplasia. Because of increased thickness of the endometrium, the blood supply to the superficial layers will be insufficient, and eventually sloughing will occur and bleeding will ensue. These patients can have various patterns of bleeding, including continuous bleeding, intermittent bleeding, premenstrual bleeding as well as heavy menstrual flow. This will be disturbing to the patient socially, and it may also lead to hypochromic anemia if untreated.

The underlying etiology of such a condition is the presence of a small number of follicles in the ovary which are resistant to the effect of gonadotropins. Ovulation will then be irregular or deficient, leading to decreased progesterone secretion.

The workup of these patients should include a complete pelvic examination to rule out any organic pelvic pathology, such as cervical polyps, tumors of the cervix, leiomyomata (fibroids) of the uterus or ovarian neoplasms. If pelvic examination is difficult due to obesity, pelvic ultrasound evaluation is necessary to rule out pelvic tumors. It is also important for the treating physician to check a quantitative B-human chorionic gonadotropin (B–HCG) assay to rule out pregnancy and its complications.

Once organic factors have been ruled out, the most probable etiology for the bleeding is anovulation, and it is called dysfunctional uterine bleeding. It is essential in these cases also to obtain an endometrial biopsy. This can usually be done in the office with the use of a pipelle sampler, which will get an adequate amount of endometrium for the pathologist to evaluate the condition of the endometrium. Frequently, the pathology evaluation will be in the form of proliferative endometrium. Rarely, it might show certain elements of cystic hyperplasia or atypia.

Thyroid screening, serum prolactin levels and serum testosterone levels should be obtained as well, to rule out any endocrinopathies. If these are present, specific management to correct these endocrine problems is in order. Rarely, coagulation defects might be encountered in the form of mild forms of von Willebrand's disease or idiopathic thrombocytopenia.

Most of these cases of dysfunctional uterine bleeding will respond very well to progestogen treatment in a cyclic fashion for ten days each cycle. Another acceptable treatment is to use low-dose oral contraceptives. Both these lines of treatment will prevent proliferative and hyperplastic changes of the endometrium, and will lead to regular endometrial shedding. Anemia will thus be avoided in these patients.

If adequate endocrine treatment has been implemented and there are no other endocrine or hematologic abnormalities, most of these patients will respond to progestogen therapy. If there is failure to respond, these patients should have hysteroscopic evaluation of the uterine cavity to rule out endometrial polyps or submucous myomas which could be causing the problem. If these are present, they can be easily removed using laser, scissors or a resectoscope, depending on the size of these lesions as well as the expertise of the gynecologist. If the patient fails to respond to these measures, the gynecologist may counsel the patient for either endometrial ablation or hysterectomy.

There is always a debate between those who favor endometrial ablation and those who favor hysterectomy. This is related to cost, recovery and patient wishes. Patients should be properly and adequately counselled on the advantages and disadvantages and complications associated with each procedure.[10] Recently, psychiatric and psychosocial effects of both procedures have been evaluated. Mental state, marital relationships, and psychosocial and sexual adjustment were not different in the hysterectomy and endometrial ablation groups of patients.[11]

The standard of care for patients undergoing hysterectomy has been very well addressed in the literature. However, the long-term follow-up of patients with endometrial ablation needs to be assessed carefully. The procedure of endometrial ablation may be associated with acute complications such as hemorrhage, uterine perforation, fluid overload and air embolism. In the follow-up of these patients, several pregnancies and cases of endometrial carcinomas have been reported.[12–15] In a recent large series of endometrial ablation cases, the authors demonstrated very good patient satisfaction. The mean follow-up of patients was 4.5 years, with the duration of the study about 11 years. The study shows a failure rate of 8%.[16]

It is also important to discuss the issue of hormone replacement when those patients who have received endometrial ablation reach menopause. These patients should be advised to use estrogens and progestogens to prevent endometrial cancer in the event of the presence of some endometrial tissue.[17]

Sometimes acute forms of anovulatory bleeding occur, manifesting with severe hemorrhage. These patients are usually brought to an emergency room with excessive blood loss. The pelvic examination in these patients reveals blood clots filling the vagina. Usually the cervix is closed and the uterus is normal in size. Hematologic studies usually reveal anemia with hemoglobin less than 10 mg per dL. In contrast to the treatment of chronic anovulatory bleeding, these patients with acute blood loss should be admitted to the hospital. The immediate treatment includes resuscitation of the blood loss by giving at least 2 units of red blood cells. Acute bleeding has been found to respond adequately to intravenous estrogen treatment in the form of Premarin, 25 mg every four to six hours for 24 to 48 hours. The patient is then put on oral Premarin, 2.5 mg daily, plus 10 mg of Provera daily for three weeks. The bleeding is usually well controlled in these cases of anovulatory bleeding, and following the three-week treatment, shedding of the endometrium occurs. The patients are then treated on the same lines as those with the chronic anovulatory type of bleeding which has been discussed.

Fertility potential in the perimenopause

The decline in fertility potential with aging is generally acknowledged. The classic study is that of the Hutterite population, where natural fertilization rates were documented in populations of women with no contraception use. These studies confirmed a slow decrease in fertility rates in women up to the age of 35, with a rapid decrease thereafter.[18] There are multiple factors contributing to this age-related decline, including decreasing numbers of oocytes and decreased oocyte quality, changes in fertilization and implantation, increased numbers of chromosome abnormalities contributing to increased spontaneous abortions and stillbirths, decreased coital frequency and increased reproductive tract disease. These issues are particularly important today, with increasing numbers of reproductive-aged women delaying both marriage and childbearing to seek careers.

The age-related decline in fecundity has been documented in studies where women with azospermatic husbands received artificial insemination by donor (AID). There is a decrease in both mean conception rate and cumulative success, beginning at the age of 31 and decreasing substantially after the age of 35. The conception rate after 12 cycles dropped from 74% in patients under 30, to 65% in patients of 30 to 34, and 56% in the 35 to 39 year age-group.[19]

The main factor contributing to the reduction in fecundity in aging women is thought to be the decline in ovarian quality and function with age. Numerous studies have documented the importance of the age of the oocyte, with regard to both normal fertilization and implantation, and the increased risk of chromosomal abnormalities seen in the aged oocyte. The follicular reserve is probably the main determinant of natural reproductive capability. As stated previously, with age there is a decrease in the number of follicles remaining, and of those which remain, the sensitivity to gonadotropins is reduced. The end result is oligo-ovulation.

Numerous investigators have reported an increase in pregnancy rates using donor oocyte programs. Women with ovarian failure over the age of 40 were given donor oocytes in combination with progesterone replacement to improve pregnancy rates, and concluded that poor oocyte quality was responsible for the age-related decline in female fertility. These results suggest that the endometrium retains its ability to respond to gonadal steroids and to provide a receptive environment for implantation and gestation even in older women.[20,21]

The superior pregnancy rates at all ages in oocyte donation programs suggest that the aging of nonovarian components is not as important as oocyte quality in the decreased fecundity in older patients. This data has been questioned because some studies failed to consider that significantly more embryos were transferred in donation cycles as compared with standard in vitro fertilization (IVF) cycles (4.5 versus 1) and that the large doses of progesterone given in other studies could mask underlying defects in the endometrium of the aged uterus. Other investigators contend that endometrial factors such as receptivity and uterine perfusion may play just as important a role in the process.[22,23]

The decreased receptivity may be secondary to decreased levels of progesterone receptors promoted by lower levels of estrogen receptors.[24] A decreased implantation rate occurs with aging. Endometrial biopsies performed in older women tend to show a high incidence of delayed or absent secretory maturation. This may be correctable with the addition of a progestational agent to support the endometrium.[19]

Animal studies have further supported the concept of uterine factors. Changes such as reduced density of stromal cells, increased collagen content and decreased estrogen receptors on endometrial cell surfaces have been described.[25,26] The age-related decline in endometrial receptivity may also be partially attributed to decreases in uterine perfusion.[23] There has been no conclusive evidence in human studies.

In addition to difficulties in conceiving, there is an increased potential for problems in pregnancies in the perimenopausal years. Common complications include a high miscarriage rate, preterm labor, antepartum hemorrhage, medical complications such as hypertension and diabetes, and postpartum hemorrhage.

There is an increase in the rate of spontaneous abortions in older age-groups. A large-scale retrospective study confirmed the association between maternal age and risk of miscarriage. When compared with women aged 20 years, the risk was doubled for pregnancies in women greater than 40. The relative risk of spontaneous abortion shows minimal change in women from 20 to 30 years old, but rises to 2.0 at the age of 40 and 3.0 at the age of 45.[27]

It has been suggested that much of the rise in rates of miscarriage is due to an increased number of chromosome abnormalities in the aged oocyte. The great majority of spontaneous abortions that occur after the age of 35 are due to chromosome anomalies, mainly autosomal trisomies. This risk increases with age.[28] Therefore genetic counseling is extremely important in this group of patients.

Further work has investigated the possibility of delayed or abnormal function in the fetoplacental unit contributing to an increased rate of abortion in older women. Some early losses were shown to occur after implantation was complete, and were accompanied by a delayed shift of steroidogenesis to the placenta of both estrogen and progesterone. The majority of the aborted pregnancies occurred at approximately 7 to 8 weeks, at the time when the placenta usually becomes autonomous in normal pregnancies.[29]

As women age, there is a greater likelihood for other factors that may further decrease their reproductive potential. For example, there is an increased risk of being affected by diseases such as endometriosis that may interfere with fertility. It is possible that occupational or environmental toxins may have an effect. In addition, previous or current exposure to sexually transmitted diseases may cause damaging effects.

It appears most likely that there is a combination of factors responsible for the decreased reproductive capability in older women. Perhaps a combined approach of oocyte donation with progesterone replacement to increase uterine receptivity would yield the best results. This would theoretically further serve to decrease the number of miscarriages secondary to chromosomal abnormalities in the aged oocyte.

Due to previous poor pregnancy outcomes in women greater than 40, physicians were somewhat hesitant to use assisted reproductive techniques and/or specialized surgical techniques to improve fertility potential in these patients. Experience with gamete intrafallopian transfer (GIFT) in women aged 40 and older has demonstrated a pregnancy rate of 9.6% per transfer, compared to a 27.3% clinical pregnancy rate per transfer in women less than 40.[30]

The IVF success rates in the past have decreased with age, especially in patients over 40. Even with modern techniques of ovulation induction and retrieval, pregnancy rates are still disappointingly low (22% per transfer).[31] This percentage is lower in older patients. With the use of donor oocytes, the success rate of IVF may be improved. Assisted hatching techniques used in combination with IVF may enhance both rates of implantation and delivery rates in the older population.[32] Thus, although assisted reproductive techniques may in fact offer successful therapy to older patients, it is important to counsel appropriately so that the patient will understand that these techniques may not completely overcome the effects on fertility of aging.

Obesity

Obesity during perimenopausal years is a serious problem both medically and socially. The prevalence of obesity in the United States is on the rise from approximately 10% to 12% about 15 years ago to 20% to 30% at present. Frequently, women at the perimenopausal stage present to their primary care physicians during a checkup complaining of small amounts of weight gain. Since this may not cause any serious medical problems, it may not be seen as that big an issue by the health care professional. However, to the patient it can be very disturbing as it is considered disfiguring to her body image.

The etiology of weight gain in perimenopausal years is not well understood. Several factors are involved, including genetic predisposition, changes in metabolism and social factors such as socioeconomic, work-related and familial stresses. Often a combination of all these factors plays a role. It is also a known fact that weight maintenance is a balance between caloric intake and expenditure. Calorie requirements are known to decrease very slightly with each menstrual period. During the perimenopausal years, the association between normal caloric intake and less caloric expenditure due to inactivity and lack of exercise definitely results in an increase in weight.

The following diagnostic methods are used for the evaluation of obesity. One of the methods is the use of the body mass index (BMI). This is calculated from the weight of the individual in kilograms divided by the height in meters squared. There are different cutoffs for what is considered normal. Generally a BMI of 19.8 to 26 is considered to be normal, while 26 or above is considered to be obesity. The World Health Organization considers obesity to be a BMI over 28.6. The National Center for Health Statistics has defined overweight as a BMI of 27.3 or more in women, and severe overweight is considered to be a BMI of 32.3 or more in women.[33]

The other commonly used diagnostic index was published in 1983 by the Metropolitan Life Insurance Company, which created tables based on height and weight. Using these charts, individuals who weigh 20% or more than the ideal body weight for their height are considered to be obese.

It is well recognized that women have a greater prevalence of obesity than men. This may be partially attributed to a lower basal resting metabolic rate (BMR). The BMR is the energy expended by a person resting in bed under fasting conditions. With aging, there is a decrease in the resting metabolic rate. As such, with no change in eating behavior or lifestyle, the older individual is destined to gain weight. It has been theorized that the peri- and postmenopausal increase in weight gain among women is in part due to a loss of the increase in the metabolic rate which is normally associated with the luteal phase of the menstrual cycle.[34]

There is an increase in body mass index with age. This is mainly due to an increase in body fat, because skeletal and lean body mass tend to decrease with age. The decrease in lean body mass starts in the perimenopausal years and continues to a great extent in the postmenopausal years. The use of hormone replacement therapy tends to improve the skeletal mass but has no demonstrable effect on lean body mass and fat content. Therefore diet and exercise programs should be suggested to women in order to prevent lean body mass loss and to decrease fat mass.

The genetic basis with regard to obesity has been researched in twin studies. Following twins who were reared apart, the incidence of obesity and overweight was similar regardless of their upbringing. The similarity was stronger between monozygotic twins than dizygotic twins. This points to a strong hereditary component of body mass index which exerts its effect with little or no influence from childhood environment. This link is further confirmed by adoptive studies which supported a relationship between overweight and biologic, not adoptive parents. This data cannot completely erase the importance of environment, however, as all children were raised in a relatively similar environment where food is plentiful.[35,36]

Weight early in life appears to have a strong association with later obesity. Independent of other factors, infant weight correlates strongly with adult weight. Infants who are greater than the 90th percentile at some point during the first six months of life are 2.6 times more likely to develop obesity than infants of average and light weight. Furthermore, adolescents who are overweight have an increased risk of later morbidity and mortality from coronary heart disease, atherosclerosis and arthritis. This is thought to be secondary to deposition of central body fat stores occurring in adolescence, affecting both blood pressure and lipoprotein profile.[37,38]

The treating physician should be aware of some of the medical problems associated with obesity. Hypertension is strongly associated with obesity. According to the second national health and examination survey between 1976 and 1989 in the United States, the prevalence of hypertension among overweight adults was found to be 2.9 times that of nonoverweight adults. The reason for the association between obesity and hypertension is multifactorial. This includes decreased renal filtration surface which may lead to renal sodium retention, increased insulin resistance with consequent hyperinsulinemia, and enhancement of tubular reabsorption of sodium. Increased plasma renin activity has been shown to be present in obese women.[39,40]

Obesity is also known to lead to changes in lipid metabolism, including a decrease in high-density lipoprotein cholesterol and an increase in low-density lipoprotein cholesterol. There is also an increase in lipoprotein lipase activity, which will lead to an increase in triglycerides.[41]

The distribution of body fat may be important in terms of risk for certain diseases. There may be more adverse effects associated with upper-body obesity such as increased insulin resistance and hyperinsulinemia. These patients have been shown to have more insulin resistance than equally obese patients with predominantly lower body fat.[42]

Hypertension, changes in the lipid metabolism and changes in insulin resistance all predispose to coronary heart disease. Both the Framingham study and the Los Angeles heart study noted a strong association between body weight and coronary artery disease. Hypertension is also known to increase the incidence of stroke.[43]

The risk of development of diabetes mellitus, gall bladder disease and respiratory disease is also increased with obesity. Studies have also reported significant increases in endometrial, cervical, ovarian and breast cancers in overweight women.

Treatment of obesity has been disappointing in the past, in part due to an incomplete understanding of the causes behind it. Permanent reversal of obesity occurs in less than 10% of patients over a ten-year period. Unrealistic expectations often lead to disappointments that further impair the weight-loss process. Proper counseling before any weight-loss program is necessary to provide guidance and set reasonable long-term goals.

The most highly recommended diet combines balanced nutrition with a program of gradual weight reduction. Crash diets are generally not successful in sustaining long-term weight loss. Important characteristics of a healthy diet include adequate nutrition, restriction of fat intake and low alcohol intake. The diet should be acceptable to the patient, with room for variation and modifications. The basic concept behind weight loss is that the diet must require less energy than is required on a daily basis to maintain body weight.

The method of dieting should be combined with a regular schedule of exercise to promote physical fitness. This is particularly important in the perimenopausal period, when loss of estrogen may contribute to bone loss. Weight-bearing activity is known to counter some of the effects of the hypoestrogenic state. Exercise also increases insulin sensitivity and thus may play an important role in combating other mechanisms, as mentioned above.

In the treatment of obesity, physicians may occasionally turn to drug therapy in a combined approach of diet and medical treatment. Most commonly prescribed are the anorectics, such as fenfluramine. Numerous studies evaluating the usefulness of this drug have indeed shown increased weight loss when compared with placebo.[44] However, long-term weight loss may not be very different. Some argue that the risks associated with such drug therapies do not outweigh the benefits.

Psychosocial and sexual issues

Along with the physical changes associated with the perimenopause is a large array of psychosocial symptoms. These symptoms may be quite distressing to the patient. These include, but are not limited to, hot flashes, joint pains, aches in the neck and skull, cold sweats and increased forgetfulness. Some women complain of having a pounding heart, constipation and fatigue. Contradicting common opinion, menopause has not been shown to be associated with depressive symptoms or crying spells.

Studies of these symptoms have shown that low levels of estrogen are associated with hot flashes. Lower estrogen levels were also found in patients who reported headaches, numbness and tingling, and dizzy spells. Thus it is logical to assume that the biological characteristics of the perimenopause may be associated with decreases in estrogen.[45]

Another important issue in the perimenopause is sexuality. Unfortunately, this topic may often go unaddressed. Vaginal dryness interfering with sexual activity may be a common complaint in the perimenopause, but patients are often embarrassed to bring up this topic on their own. This dryness may lead to severe dyspareunia, bleeding, vaginitis, anorgasmia or sexual aversion. It is important for the physician to bring up these issues, so that appropriate examination and treatment options can be adequately addressed to improve quality of life.[46]

Sexually transmitted disease (STD) also needs to be addressed. In the United States, although there has been a general decline in rates of STDs, there continues to be a large amount of infection, especially in the inner-city minority populations. The most common STD is chlamydia, although the incidence of this is also decreasing. In addition, the incidence of STDs continues to be high in developing countries, posing a major public health concern. With the exclusion of HIV, sexually transmitted diseases are the second most common cause of healthy life lost, exceeded only by maternal morbidity and mortality.

Although most diagnoses of STDs lie within younger populations, diagnosis of STD in the older age-group is not an infrequent occurrence. Appropriate prevention strategies that aim at early diagnosis and reducing the risk of acquiring STDs may often fail to target this older population. The most serious complications associated with STDs include ectopic pregnancy, pelvic inflammatory disease, decreased fertility and cervical cancer associated with HPV (Human papilloma virus). With the predicted increase in the number of elderly women, these issues may become increasingly important.

Infections due to chlamydia have become the most prevalent of sexually transmitted diseases. Mandated national reporting started in 1994. These infections are often responsible for serious reproductive tract complications, including pelvic inflammatory disease, ectopic pregnancy and infertility. Although the highest incidence is seen in the younger population, clinical manifestations relating to later infertility and pain secondary to pelvic adhesions may play an important role later in life.

In 1994, chlamydial infections as reported were found for the first time to exceed those due to gonorrhea. Most of these infections occurred in the younger age-groups. Among women tested in family planning clinics, the percent of positivity showed a progressively decreasing incidence as age increased. This difference was particularly significant when the younger age-groups, under 19, were compared with women 30 years of age and older.

With age-specific rates of gonorrhea, there is also a large decrease in incidence as age increases. The incidence appears fairly uniform among women over 30 years old, although there is a slight decline when comparing those aged 30 to 34 years of age to those 35 to 39, and to those 40 to 44 years old. The reported rate per 100,000 in women between 40 and 44 years of age was 27.6 in 1994, as compared to 92.7 in the 15- to 19-year-old age-group. The decline continues down to 9.0 per 100,000 for women aged 45 to 54. The most impressive decrease in the incidence of gonorrhea has occurred in the under-19 age-group. The incidence in the 30-and-above age-group has appeared relatively constant.

As with gonorrhea, there has been a progressive decline in the incidence of both primary and secondary syphilis. There was a small increase in cases around 1990, but this has progressively declined to the lowest number of reported cases since 1977. As with the other STDs, the age-specific incidence decreases dramatically as age increases. Rates per 100,000 in 1994 were highest in the 20 to 24 age-group, at 24.2, decreasing to 2.5 in the 45 to 54 age-group.

In terms of HIV, in the US 10% of AIDS cases are reported in persons 50 years of age and older. Only 1% occur in those older than 65.[47,48] In conclusion, perimenopausal women should be counselled in regard to the prevalence of these sexually transmitted diseases and the use of conventional barrier methods for protection.

REFERENCES

1 Khaw KT: Epidemiology of the menopause. *Br Med Bull* 48(2): 249,1992.

2 Aiman J: A history of human fertility. In *Infertility: Diagnosis and Management*, ed. Aiman J. New York: Springer–Verlag, 1984, pp. 1–6.

3 US Bureau of the Census: *Statistical Abstract of the United States, 1990*, 100th edition. Washington DC.

4 Speroff I: A clinician's approach to therapy during a woman's transition years. *Contemporary OB/ GYN*, August 1991, 65–68.

5 Ebbiary A, Lenton EA, Cooke ID: Hypothalamic–pituitary aging: Progressive increase in FSH and LH concentration throughout the reproductive life in regularly menstruating women. *Clin Endocrinol* 41(2): 199,1994.

6 Cocchi D: Age–related alterations in gonadotropin, adrenocorticotropin, and growth hormone secretion. *Aging* 4(2): 103,1992.

7 Vihko KK, Kiyansuu E, Morsky P, Huhtaniemi I, Punnonen R: Gonadotropins and gonadotropin receptors during the perimenopause. *Europ J Endocrinol* 134(3): 357,1996.

8 Gosden RG, Faddy MJ: Ovarian aging, follicular depletion, and steroidogenesis. *Exp Gerontol* 29(3–4): 265,1994.

9 Wentz AC: Abnormal uterine bleeding. In *Novak's Textbook of Gynecology*, Howard W Jones III, Anne Colston Wentz, Lonnie S. Burnett, eds., Baltimore MD; Williams and Wilkins, pp. 378–396,1988.

10 Pinion SB, Parkin DE, Abromovich DR, Naji A, Alexander DA, Russell IT, Kitcher HC: Randomized trial of hysterectomy, endometrial ablation, and transcervical endometrial resection for dysfunctional uterine bleeding. *Brit Med J* 309(6960): 979,1994.

11 Alexander DA, Naji AA, Pinion SB, Hollison J, Kitchner HC, Parkin DE, Abramovich DR, Russell IT: Randomized trial comparing hysterectomy with endometrial ablation for dysfunctional uterine bleeding: Psychiatric and psychosocial aspects. *Brit Med J* 312(7026): 280,1996.

12 Ramey JW, Koonings PP, Given FT Jr, Acosta AA: The process of carcinogenesis for endometrial adenocarcinoma could be short: Development of a malignancy after endometrial ablation. *Am J Obstet Gynecol* 170(5pt1): 1370,1994.

13 Copperman AB, DeCherney AH, Olive DL: A case of endometrial cancer following endometrial ablation for dysfunctional uterine bleeding. *Obstet Gynecol* 82(4pt2 suppl): 640,1993.

14 McLucas B: Pregnancy after endometrial ablation. A case report. *J Reprod Med* 40(3): 237,1995.

15 Baumann R, Owerdieck W, Reck G: Pregnancy following sterilization and endometrial resection. *Geburtshilfe und Frauenheilkunde* 54(4): 246,1994.

16 Baggish MS, Sze EH: Endometrial ablation: A series of 568 patients treated over an 11-year period. *Am J Obstet Gynecol* 174(3): 908,1996.

17 Istre O, Holm-Nielsen P, Bourne T, Forman A: Hormone replacement therapy after transcervical resection of the endometrium. *Obstet Gynecol* 88: 767,1996.

18 Tietze C: Reproductive span and rate of reproduction among Hutterite women, *Fertil Steril* 8: 89,1957.

19 Schwartz D, Mayaux MJ: Female fecundity as a function of age: Results of artificial insemination in 2193 nulliparous women with azoospermic husbands. Federation CECOS. *N Engl J Med* 306: 404,1982.

20 Sauer MV, Paulson RJ, Lobo RA: A preliminary report on oocyte donation extending reproductive potential to women over 40. *N Engl J Med* 323: 1157,1990.

21 Navot D, Drews MR, Bergh PA, Guzman I, Karstaedt A, Scott RT, Garrisi GJ, Hofmann GE: Age-related decline in female fertility is not due to diminished capacity of the uterus to sustain embryo implantation. *Fertil Steril* 61: 97,1994.

22 Yaron Y, Botchan A, Amit A, Kogosowski A, Yovel I, Lessing JB: Endometrial receptivity: The age-related decline in pregnancy rates and the effect of ovarian function. *Fertil Steril* 60: 314,1993.

23 Goswamy RK, Williams G, Steptoe PC: Decreased uterine perfusion; a cause of infertility. *Hum Reprod* 3: 955,1988.

24 Meldrum DR: Female reproductive aging–ovarian and uterine factors. *Fertil Steril* 59: 1,1993.

25 Craig SS, Jollie WP: Age changes in density of endometrial stromal cells of the rat. *Exp Gerontol* 20: 93,1985.

26 Han Z, Kokkonen GC, Roth GS: Effect of aging on populations of estrogen receptor-containing cells in the rat uterus. *Exp Cell Res* 180: 234,1989.

27 Risch HA, Weiss NS, Clarke EA, Miller AB: Risk factors for spontaneous abortion and its recurrence. *Am J Epidemiol* 128: 420,1988.

28 Warburton D, Kline J, Stein Z, Strobino B: Cytogenetic abnormalities in spontaneous abortions of recognized conceptions. In Porter IH, ed., *Perinatal Genetics: Diagnosis and Treatment*, New York: Academic Press, 1986, p 133.

29 Cano F, Simon C, Remohi J, Pellicer A: Effect of age on the female reproductive system: Evidence for a role of uterine senescence in the decline in female fecundity. *Fertil Steril* 64(3): 584,1995.

30 Penzias AS, Thompson IE, Alper MM, Oskowitz SP, Berger MJ: Successful use of gamete intrafallopian transfer does not reverse the decline in fertility in women over 40 years of age. *Obstet Gynecol* 77: 37,1991.

31 IVF-ET Registry: In vitro fertilization – embryo transfer (IVF-ET) in the United States: 1990 results from the IVF-ET registry. *Fertil Steril* 57: 15,1992.

32 Schoolcraft UB, Schlenken T et al.: In vitro fertilization in women aged 40 and older: The impact of assisted hatching. *J Assist Repro Genetics* 12(9): 581,1995.

33 Williamson DF: Descriptive epidemiology of body weight and weight change in U.S. adults. *Ann Intern Med* 119: 646–649,1993.

34 Ferraro R, Lillioja S, Fontvielle A-M, Rising R, Bogardus C, Ravussin E: Lower sedentary metabolic rate in women compared with men. *J Clin Invest* 90: 780,1992.

35 Stunkard AJ, Harris JR, Pederson NL, McClearn GE: The body-mass index of twins who have been reared apart. *New Engl J Med* 322: 461,1990.

36 Stunkard AJ, Sorenson TIA, Teasdale TW, Chakraborty R, Schull WJ, Schulsinger F: An adoptive study of human obesity. *New Engl J Med* 314: 193,1986.

37 Charney E, Goodman HC, McBride M, Lyon B, Pratt R: Childhood antecedents of adult obesity. *New Engl J Med* 295: 6,1976.

38 Must A, Jacques PF, Dallal GE, Bajema CJ, Dietz WH: Long-term morbidity and mortality of

adolescents: A follow-up of the Harvard Growth Study of 1922 to 1935. *New Engl J Med* 327: 1350,1992.

39 Pi-Sunyer FX: Medical hazards of obesity. *Ann Intern Med* 119: 655–660,1993.

40 Havlik RJ, Hubert HB, Fabsitz RR, Feinleib M: Weight and hypertension. *Ann Intern Med* 98: 855–859,1983.

41 Assman S, Schulte H: Obesity and hyperlipidemia: Results from the prospective cardiovascular munster (PROCAM) study. In Bjorn-torp P, Brodoff BN, eds. *Obesity.* New York: J.B. Lippincott, 1992, pp. 502–511.

42 Stern MP, Haffner SM: Body fat distribution and hyperinsulinemia as risk factors for diabetes and cardiovascular disease. A review. *Arteriosclerosis* 6: 123–129,1986.

43 Hubert HB, Feinleib M, McNamara PM, Castelli WP: Obesity as an independent risk factor for cardiovascular disease: A 26 year follow-up of participants in the Framingham Heart Study. *Circulation* 67: 968–977,1983.

44 Garrow JS: Treatment of obesity. *Lancet* 33: 409–413,1992.

45 Matthews KA, Wing RR, Kuller LH, Meilahn EN, Plantinga P: Influence of the perimenopause on cardiovascular risk factors and symptoms of middle-aged healthy women. *Arch Intern Med* 154: 2349–2355,1994.

46 Plumbo MA: Clinical intervention framework for a sexual complaint of the perimenopause. *J Nurse Midwifery* 39(3): 157,1994.

47 Centers for Disease Control: Cases of selected notifiable diseases, United States. *MMWR* 45(1): 13–25,1996.

48 US Department of Health and Human Services, Public Health Service. *Sexually Transmitted Diseases Surveillance, 1994.* Atlanta: Centers for Disease Control, 1995.

2

The endocrinology of the menopause

MANVINDER SINGH

Female life expectancy is approaching 80 years of age. The average age of menopause has been 50 to 51 years in the United States for the last couple of centuries. Women are now living more than one-third of their life in menopause. It is important for the clinician to understand the hormonal and physiological changes with the menopause as well as the associated psychological aspects, to be able to prevent and treat the related problems during this stage of a woman's life.

The climacterium is usually between the ages of 40 to 60 years of age. This is a period in which there is decline in fertility. There is gradual progression from the perimenopause to the postmenopausal era. The perimenopause is a period in which a woman's ovarian function regresses gradually. This process starts with luteal-phase defects, progressing to anovulation and then to complete cessation of menstruation. Women can go through periods of hypoestrogenism or periods of hyperestrogenism, causing a whole array of pathological conditions. Perimenopause is a period in which the ovarian function is slowly diminishing. This process can take up to five years. Multiple symptomatology can occur at this time, including hot flashes, menstrual-cycle aberrations and premenstrual symptoms as well. Other symptoms can also occur with associated medical ailments or with changing family dynamics such as divorce or kids entering college.

Usually, menopause sets in gradually. The early years of menopause are most notable for bone depletion with a potential for osteoporosis. This is a gradual process that takes many years. Cardiovascular disease has a much higher prevalence rate in the menopause. In fact, more women die of cardiovascular-related illnesses than any other condition. Estrogens are protective of adverse cardiovascular events in the menopause. Having benefited from high estrogen levels during their premenopausal years, women are protected from adverse cardiovascular events as compared to men.[1] Progressive hypoestrogenism after a woman is well into the menopause (10 to 20 years) can eventually lead to genital atrophy, which at times can be quite debilitating, causing vaginitis and difficulty with intercourse.

It is estimated that 30 to 40% of menopausal women have either minor or no symptoms at all. The rest of the menopausal women are symptomatic. Ten percent of these women have severe symptoms. The asymptomatic group of menopausal women need the same evaluation as the symptomatic women because they all suffer from hypoestrogenism. They all need the proper counseling for the therapeutic value of estrogen treatment. This will lead to more compliance when hormone replacement is prescribed.[2]

The endocrinological changes in the menopause are complicated by the changes that are associated with usual aging. As the ovaries are being depleted of ova, estrogen levels diminish, and menopause gradually sets in. Along with this process, numerous other diseases and ailments can occur concomitantly, confusing issues of menopause. As one ages, there is decreasing adrenal function, higher incidence of thyroid disease in the fifth decade onwards, decreasing melatonin levels and other endocrinologic changes. The clinician has to be aware of the interplay of different endocrine systems in menopause and aging, so that a patient can be assessed completely and systematically.

LIFE CYCLE OF THE OVARY

During ovarian development in the fetus, the number of oocytes increases to reach a maximum of six to seven million at about the twentieth week of gestation. The oocyte number then gradually declines to one to two million at birth. Follicular atresia continues during childhood until puberty when the number of oocytes reaches three to four hundred thousand.[3] Once the hypothalamic–pituitary–ovarian axis has been activated through a state of derepression, the pubertal process starts. Estrogen production from the ovary gradually increases as primordial follicles are stimulated to maturation and ovulation. Most women undergo three to four hundred ovulatory cycles in their lifetimes until all oocytes from the ovaries are exhausted. As one oocyte ovulates, a thousand become atretic per each cycle through a process called apoptosis.[4,5]

The ovulatory cycle is under numerous physiologic and endocrine controls. Initially, as estradiol levels become basilar, the follicle-stimulating hormone (FSH) levels start to increase with increased pulsation of gonadotropin-releasing hormone. A primordial follicle is stimulated ahead of the others and eventually becomes a dominant follicle. The dominant follicle has the highest levels of estradiol and FSH receptors. Through positive influences of estradiol, FSH receptors increase in concentration and number compared with other follicles. Thus, the dominant follicle continues to grow and other follicles become atretic. The increase in estradiol level has a negative influence on FSH levels, which decline subsequently. However, the dominant follicles continue to be stimulated because the FSH receptors concentration is still relatively high. The dominant follicle continues to increase in size to approximately 2.0 cm. in diameter, until a luteinizing hormone (LH) surge causes ovulation. Estradiol gradully increases from basilar levels to about 300 pg/ml prior to ovulation. Another estradiol peak is noted in the middle of the luteal phase.[6]

Inhibin from the developing follicles also has negative feedback influence on the FSH levels.[7,8] Inhibin concentration has been known to diminish in the developing follicles of older women, further attesting to the incompetency of oocytes in the older women, as discussed in the chapter on perimenopause.[9] For this reason, FSH levels at days one to three of the cycle are relatively high in the perimenopause and can be used as a marker for ovarian reserve.[10,11]

Eventually, as a result of depleted oocytes from both ovaries, no further follicular development occurs; FSH levels will rise ten- to twentyfold and LH will rise threefold. These levels remain high until the third year into the menopause. The FSH levels are higher than LH levels primarily because the half life of LH (half an hour) is eight times less than FSH (four hours). In the menopause, the FSH and LH hormones have an increased carbohydrate component which is less biologically active when compared to premenopausal FSH and LH. This fact may be due to a low estrogen state.[12]

ENDOCRINOLOGY OF THE MENOPAUSAL OVARY

The menopausal ovary contains very few to no ova. Hence the production of ovarian estrogens is almost nonexistent. Testosterone production, on the other hand, continues, because the stroma of the ovary is conserved. Sex-hormone-binding globulin (SHBG) is decreased in the menopause due to the marked reduction of ovarian estradiol production. Because of these facts, numerous pathophysiologic effects can be seen in the menopause.

A very elaborate study by Goswamy and colleagues found that the average size of right and left ovaries in 2,246 postmenopausal women studied was 3.6 mL.[13] Factors which influence the size include years since menopause, weight and parity. As few or no follicles are present in the ovary and virtually no granulosa cells, only ovarian androgens continue to be produced in the menopause, because the stroma contains theca cells. The main estrogen in the menopause is estrone and not 17 β-estradiol as seen in the premenopausal women. Estrone is derived predominantly from aromatization of adrenal androstenedione. The daily production of estrone is also related to body weight and age. There is no significant decrease of estrogen production in castrated postmenopausal women as compared to castrated premenopausal women. When glucocorticoids are given to postmenopausal women, there is a significant lowering of estrogens, indicating an adrenal source of estrogens in the menopause. Gradient studies have shown no difference in ovarian veins versus arteries in 17 β-estradiol concentrations, as opposed to a significant gradient difference noted with testosterone and androstenedione in the menopause. Androstenedione can be peripherally converted to either testosterone or estradiol and estrone.[14,15] Some degree of aromatization may occur in the postmenopausal ovary, although this is considered to be insignificant.

The ovary retains its ability to continue androgen production. 3 β-hydroxysteroid dehydrogenase activity is still present, as noted by histochemical studies.[16] In vitro studies show that when labeled pregnenolone is added to strips of ovarian stroma, labeled progesterone, dehydroepiandrosterone and testosterone are obtained,[15] indicating that the postmenopausal ovary is capable of steroidogenesis to some degree. Human chorionic gonadotropin (HCG) causes increased cyclic adenosine monophosphate levels in postmenopausal ovarian strips in vitro.[17] This further proves that the elevated gonadotropins can drive the ovary to continue to produce androgens.[18] In fact, on rare occasions menopausal ovaries can become hyperplastic or hyperthecotic, and women bearing these ovaries can develop significant manifestations of hirsutism and virilization with testosterone levels in the tumor range (that is, greater than 200 ng/dL). Medullary components such as the hilar cell are also active, whereas the vessels in the medulla are atrophic. Hilar cells respond to HCG even more so than the stroma. Hilar cell tumors are occasionally seen in menopausal women with signs of hirsutism and virilization.[19–22] These tumors can be quite small and difficult to diagnose.

Androstenedione production from the menopausal ovary is half as great as it is premenopausally. In the menopause, most of the androstenedione is derived from the adrenal gland, unlike the premenopausal state, where half the androstenedione is adrenal in origin and half is ovarian in origin. There is a 20% reduction of androstenedione from the adrenal gland once menopause has set in. In total, the ratio of adrenal to ovarian androstenedione contribution in the menopause is 4:1.[23] Further support for this premise is noted by the fact that corticotropin causes marked androstenedione increase, whereas HCG does not.[24]

Testosterone production decreases in the menopause to a lesser degree than does androstenedione production. The ovarian production of testosterone is maintained, whereas production of testosterone from other sites is diminished. There is a 50% reduction in testosterone levels after oophorectomy.[25] The loss of ovarian androstenedione production in oophorectomized women does not account for the testosterone production loss due to conversion of androstenedione to testosterone, because the amount of androstenedione of ovarian origin is minimal.

Gonadotropins are able to bind to menopausal ovaries, as demonstrated by autoradiography studies using I-125 labeled gonadotropins, and measurable amounts of androstenedione, estradiol and progesterone are increased with administration of gonadotropins. Histochemical evidence of steroidogenesis is noted when human chorionic gonadotropin is injected *in vivo*.[26–28] Treatment with gonadotropin-releasing hormone (GnRH) analog in postmenopausal women causes decreased testosterone, estradiol and androstenedione levels. Estrone levels remain unchanged as there is no effect on adrenal androstenedione production and hence on its conversion.[29]

In summary, the postmenopausal ovary is primarily an androgen-producing gland (Figure 2.1). Estrogens are produced by the aged ovary, but only minimally; therefore, this does not produce any physiologic effect. The main estrogen is derived from the conversion of androstenedione to estrone. This conversion is through a process of peripheral aromatization. Most of the androstenedione is produced from the adrenal gland. FSH and LH levels are high as a result of hypoestrogenism. Numerous pathophysiologic effects are pronounced as a result of hypoestrogenism, such as hot flashes, osteoporosis, cardiovascular problems, vaginal dryness and others.

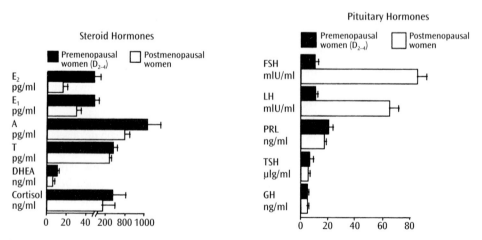

Figure 2.1 *Hormone levels before and after menopause. E_2 = estradiol; E_1 = estrone; A = androstenedione; T = testosterone; DHEA = dehydroepiandrosterone; PRL = prolactin; GH = growth hormone. Reproduced with permission of Yen SSC. Reproduced with permission from the* Journal of Reproductive Medicine 1977; 18: 287–96.

ENDOCRINOLOGY OF THE HOT FLASH

The hot flash is a warm sensation starting from the back of the head or neck and disseminating throughout the body, accompanied by intense heat. The hot flash can be rather troublesome, causing sleep disturbances, irritability and anxiety. The incidence of the hot flash in the menopause is up to 70%.[30] It tends to occur more often in warm climates, and is either more severe or more noticeable at night. At times it awakens patients from sleep with profuse sweating.[31] The rate of hot flashes declines over age in most women. It can be persistent in some women for many years.

The etiology of the hot flash still remains a mystery. Withdrawal of estrogens can consistently cause hot flashes in most individuals. Individuals who have been hypoestrogenic for their entire lifetime, such as patients with Turner's syndrome and patients with lifelong hypothalamic amenorrhea, do not suffer from hot flashes. Individuals who have stopped estrogen replacement therapy, have recently been surgically castrated or have been treated with GnRH agonists have hot flashes.

It therefore seems that the estrogens convey some developed effect which, after withdrawal, causes a shift in thermoregulatory processes within the hypothalamus. The hypothalamus is considered to be the starting point from which the hot flash starts.

Obese women can be protected from the development of hot flashes because they have high estrone production through peripheral aromatization of androstenedione.[32] There is also more free estrogen available as SHBG is decreased.[33]

LH pulsations are associated with the hot flash. It is no longer thought that the LH pulses cause the hot flash because studies indicate that the LH pulse actually occurs after the start of the flash. Women who are given HCG in ovulation induction do not have hot flashes. Women who have had their pituitary gland removed can still have hot flashes.[34]

Estrogen induces hypothalamic opioid activity. The loss of this opioid activity may cause the thermodysregulation seen with the hot flash. Estrogen's thermoregulatory effect may also be mediated by norepinephrine.[35] Estrogen stimulates tyrosine hydroxylase activity, which increases norepinephrine.[36] Estrogens can decrease the degradation of norepinephrine. Estrogens also augment norepinephrine release and inhibit norepinephrine reuptake.[37] Estrogen can increase hypothalamic $alpha_2$ postsynaptic receptors.[38] These actions serve to enhance $alpha_2$ adrenergic activity (Figure 2.2). Vasomotor flashes may be a result of

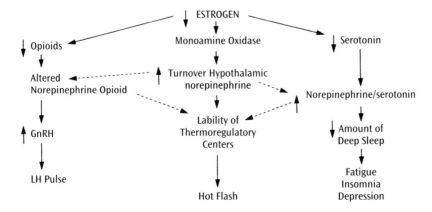

Figure 2.2 *Possible mechanisms of central nervous system change in climacteric women. Reproduced with permission from Hammond CB. The climacteric. In: Danforth's obstetrics and gynecology. 7th ed. Philadelphia: Lippincott, 1994.*

reduced alpha$_2$ adrenergic activity. For this reason alpha$_2$ adrenergic agents such as clonidine are used to retard hot flashes[39,40] and alpha$_2$ adrenergic antagonists such as yohimbine
cause hot flashes.[41]

OSTEOPOROSIS

Osteoporosis affects 20 million women in the United States. Most commonly, postmenopausal women are affected. There are 1.5 million hip, wrist and spine fractures annually.
Spine fractures are the most commonly associated with osteoporosis.[42] In fact, 25% of
women greater than 60 years of age have spinal compression factors. At 75 years of age and
above, 50% of women have spinal fractures. Hip fractures are less common than spinal
fractures; however, one in six women with hip fractures dies within three months of having
had the hip fracture.

Therefore, it is important to control osteoporosis in any given patient. Women live
longer and a third of their life is in a hypoestrogenic stage. Osteoporosis can occur in any
particular bone. The more common areas of fracture include the vertebrae, the hip (at the
femoral neck or intertrochanteric region) and the wrist (also termed Colles' fracture). At
present the three major osteoporotic fracture types cost the United States 15 to 30 billion
dollars per year.[43] As the population ages, these figures will steadily increase. The reasons
for bone loss are not only hypoestrogenism but also include decreasing physical activity and
inadequate calcium and vitamin D intake. Inadequate vitamin D intake may be more
problematic in areas where there is decreased sunlight because the active vitamin D
compound is produced less in such conditions (Figure 2.3). Increased intake of alcohol
or caffeine, cigarette smoking or glucocorticoid use can exacerbate the disease process.
There can also be a genetic predisposition for the occurrence of osteoporosis.[44]

Sex, race, nutrition and overall health influence osteoporosis. Black people are less prone
than Caucasians to having osteoporosis. Subsequent rate of bone resorption is noted to be a
factor. Bone mass declines after peak because of remodeling imbalance. There is a rapid
decline of bone after menopause. Approximately 15% of bone is lost every 10 years. The risk
factors for osteoporosis include Caucasian women, a slight build and a positive family history.
Women who are overweight or obese are somewhat protected from osteoporosis because of
the higher level of estrogens that will form through peripheral conversion of androstenedione to estrone. Other risk factors can also include deficiency of estrogens early in
life with premature ovarian failure caused by radiation therapy or chemotherapy. History of
extreme exercise can also cause osteoporosis, as this also produces a hypoestrogenic state.[44]

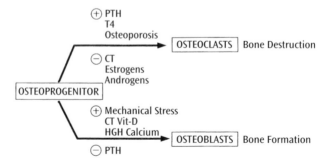

Figure 2.3 *Mechanisms of bone metabolism. PTH = parathormone; T4 = thyroxine; CT = calcitonin;
Vit-D = vitamin D; HGH = growth hormone.*

It is important to realize that the skeleton is a major target organ of estrogens. Bone remodeling is modulated by estrogens, and the hypoestrogenic state allows for further resorption of bone. This leads to a reduced skeletal mass which is accompanied by micro-architectural deterioration of bone. This ultimately predisposes the bone to fracture. The mechanism by which estrogens are involved in maintaining bone is not well understood. It is important to realize that peak bone mass occurs at age 35 and declines in subsequent years.

The clinical signs of osteoporosis can be seen in gradual loss of height, dorsal kyphosis with a dowager's hump, chronic back pain, pulmonary dysfunction, early satiety, bloating or constipation, or an atraumatic fracture. Bone mass decreases with decreasing activity, and calcium loss can occur at up to 200 mg to 300 mg per day on full bed rest. Moderate exercise has been shown to be beneficial in maintaining bone, especially with weight–bearing exercise, of at least 30 minutes three times a week. It has been quite well established that for postmenopausal women on estrogen replacement therapy, 1000 mg of calcium is needed per day, whereas for postmenopausal women not on estrogen replacement therapy, 1500 mg of calcium is needed per day. Supplementation should be started early – before reaching 35 years of age, according to some sources.[44]

For women prior to menopause, bone loss is equal to bone loss in men. On the average, men lose approximately 3% to 5% of bone per decade. After the menopause, women start to lose bone mass much more rapidly than men. Women lose approximately 2% per year for up to the first 10 years. The largest loss occurs in the early postmenopausal years.[44] Accelerated bone loss in women versus men explains why women are more prone to osteoporosis and related injuries.

Other factors to keep in mind are that the bone is an interactive tissue and not stagnant. There is constant building and breaking down of bone. The osteoblasts are one type of bone cells and are noted to be multinucleated giant cells that measure 20 to 100 microns in diameter. They are found in areas of bone which are undergoing resorption, called lacunae of howship. Osteoclasts increase activity in response to parathyroid hormone. Their activity is decreased with calcitonin. Increased osteoclastic activity is noted when there are high levels of urinary hydroxyproline and pyridinoline. Osteoblasts are found in areas of bone remodeling and can secrete collagen and other substances that make bone. Osteocalcin is a marker of osteoblastic activity. The hormones PTH and 1-25 Vitamin D stimulate bone resorption, and receptors for both hormones are found on osteoblasts. Calcitonin is another hormone that can affect bone formation. It is produced by the parafollicular cells in the thyroid gland, and production is decreased by increased calcium concentration. Calcitonin inhibits osteoclastic activity, causes an increase in bone formation and also decreases the excretion of calcium by the kidneys. Calcitonin is available for treatment of osteoporosis in nasal spray and injection forms.

CARDIOVASCULAR DISEASE IN THE MENOPAUSE

Cardiovascular disease remains the leading cause of death in American women. The incidence of cardiovascular disease rises sharply after menopause. Having benefited from a high-estrogen state, premenopausal women are protected from cardiovascular disease, as opposed to women in the menopause, who are in a low-estrogen state. Menopausal women on estrogen replacement therapy are also protected from cardiovascular disease. Obesity and cigarette smoking have clouded the issues of cardiovascular disease in menopause. It is apparent that obesity and cigarette smoking contribute to cardiovascular disease and that smoking is a more important risk factor for cardiovascular disease than is obesity. In one study in which natural menopause and heart disease were examined, the risk of calcifications in the aorta was greater in the postmenopausal woman than in premenopausal women, with a relative risk of 3.4 (95% confidence intervals of 1.2 to 9.7).[45] The risk of cardiovascular disease increases in women who are not using estrogen treatment. Approximately 23% of women have a risk of dying of ischemic heart disease. This is dramatically high as compared to breast cancer in which the percentage risk is 4%, osteoporotic factors, in which the percentage risk is 2.5% and reproductive tract malignancies, in which the percentage risk is 2%.[46]

Obesity is an independent risk factor because of its relationship to hypertension, hyperlipidemia, insulin resistance and diabetes mellitus. Android obesity, or centralized obesity as seen in men, is a high risk factor as well. There is a strong association between android obesity and insulin resistance and hyperinsulinemia. The higher the total cholesterol level and the higher the low-density lipoprotein (LDL) levels, the greater the risk factors for coronary artery disease. Hypertension, which includes elevated systolic and diastolic blood pressures, is also a known risk factor. Hyperinsulinemia, insulin resistance and chronic hyperglycemia attribute to coronary artery disease through hyperlipidemia. Controlling these can control or decrease coronary artery disease. Cigarette smoking in a dose-dependent manner has been shown to worsen cardiovascular disease.

Estrogens are able to retard athersosclerotic processes by modifying lipid metabolism or by preventing thickening of the intimal portion of blood vessels. The hepatocytes are known to contain estrogen receptors. In the menopause, there is a decrease in turnover of LDL cholesterol and decreased production of high-density lipoprotein (HDL) cholesterol. This abnormal ratio contributes to the risk for cardiovascular disease. When women are given estrogen therapy, they are able to reverse the ratio of LDL to HDL, thereby decreasing their chances of cardiovascular-related problems. The percentage decrease of LDL cholesterol has been noted to be approximately 15%, whereas the percentage increase of HDL has been noted to be on the average 11%.[47] Progestogens combined with estrogen replacement therapy seem to negate some of the effects that estrogen has on the LDL/HDL ratio. Atherosclerotic disease is better predicted by hypertriglyceridemia and low LDH cholesterol levels in women than in men. Atherosclerosis is also associated with hypertension, obesity, diabetes and insulin resistance. Estrogen benefits include increasing the levels of apoprotein A1 and lowering apoprotein B and fibrinogen levels. Estrogens can also be considered as antioxidants and protect the integrity of the endothelial cell from potential injury. Estrogens can inhibit adhesion formation in artherosclerosis and platelet aggregation. This ultimately retards the formation of a thrombus. These, along with other effects, account for the 56% reduction of coronary artery disease. In patients with coronary artery disease, it is noted that the endothelium does not respond normally to acetylcholine. In estrogen-deficient animals, acetylcholine causes coronary vasoconstriction, whereas in estrogenized animals it causes the opposite effect.[48] Furthermore, in women having cardiac catheterizations, infusion of ethinyl estradiol decreases basal coronary arterial tone in acutely attenuated, acetylcholine-induced constriction in these vessels.[47] Estradiol can restore the vasodilation response prior to administration of acetylcholine.[50] When estradiol is given sublingually before treadmill testing, fewer ischemic episodes were noted.[51] The estrogen-mediated vasodilatation is probably mediated by nitric oxide.[50] Hormone replacement therapy increases circulating nitric oxide levels in postmenopausal women.[53] Estrogens can further induce arteriolar relaxation in the vessels without endothelium. Estradiol receptors have been found in smooth muscles of coronary arteries.[54] It has been shown that artherosclerotic lesions can regress, and this implies that estrogens have a profound effect on the circulatory system throughout the body.[53]

For all these reasons, estrogens should be used for prevention of heart disease in postmenopausal women. The direct effects of estrogen on arterial walls include reduced LDL accumulation, arterial cholesterol influx and hydrolysis. In addition there is inhibition of platelet aggregation, reduced lipoprotein and induced arterial smooth-muscle proliferation. With estrogens there is reduced myointimal proliferation associated with mechanical injury or induced by stress, decreased collagen, and elastin production. Increased arterial smooth-muscle prostacyclin production and inhibition of foam cell formation are also seen with estrogens. Estrogens can also have a direct ionotropic action on the heart and can improve glucose metabolism with potential decrease in circulating insulin levels.[55]

ATROPHIC GENITAL CHANGES

Atrophy of the female genitalia is a late feature in the postmenopausal woman. The vaginal mucosa becomes thinner and loses its rugations ultimately leading to vaginitis, pruritis and considerable stenosis. Not only is the vagina affected, but the urethra and the bladder can be affected as well. Urinary incontinence, urethritis and urge incontinence can all be problems associated with mucosal thinning of the urethra and bladder, and recurrent urinary tract infections can occur. Vaginal relaxation with cystocele and rectocele, and uterine prolapse are also possible. Mild forms of genuine stress incontinence can be improved with estrogen therapy alone, as can urge incontinence and atrophic vaginitis. Estrogen receptors have been found in the external genitalia, vagina, urethra and bladder. The vulva can lose its lush appearance due to decreased fatty tissue and collagen. Lack of intercourse during the menopause is a confounding factor which can lead to significant vaginal narrowing and loss of elasticity in itself. The secretions of the vagina are also lost, and intercourse can be painful. Sexual dysfunction can be a major problem in older women. Estrogen replacement therapy can correct all these atrophic changes, leading to improvement or cure of all these manifestations.[56–59]

NEUROENDOCRINOLOGY RELATED TO THE POSTMENOPAUSAL WOMAN

In the central nervous system, the greatest numbers of estrogen receptors are found in the pituitary, hypothalamus, limbic system, forebrain and cerebral cortex.[60] The limbic system can be influenced by circulating estrogen. Estrogens can alter a number of neurotransmitters, including serotonin.[61] All of these facts show how estrogen could potentially affect mood. It is possible that a decrease in estrogen levels could therefore alter mood in the menopausal period. The hippocampus is critically important to learning and memory and also contains estrogen receptors. Estrogens increase choline acetyl transferase activity and thereby increase acetylcholine, which is the agent thought to be needed for memory. Further studies are needed to elucidate how estrogens affect the central nervous system. Progestogens, on the other hand, seem to have adverse effects of depression and sedation.

THYROID CHANGES IN AGING

The clinician must be cognizant of thyroid changes occurring in the menopause. Atypical hot flashes can present as hyperthyroidism. The incidence of hypothyroidism increases in women older than 40. The incidence of this condition can be as high as 10% of such women. Thyroid problems occur four to five times more often in women than in men.

Thyroid physiology

The thyroid gland is under direct control of thyroid-stimulating hormone (TSH) produced by the pituitary gland. The pituitary gland receives hormonal influxes of thyroid releasing hormone (TRH) from the hypothalamus and releases TSH. There is a negative feedback loop in play. When the thyroid hormone T4 is elevated, this will suppress TRH and TSH. When the T4 is low, this raises TRH and TSH.

Estrogens have been known to cause an increase in responsiveness of TRH to TSH. TRH also causes an increase in prolactin (PRL) secretion. In states of overt primary hypothyroidism, prolactin levels could be elevated enough to cause galactorrhea, thereby emphasizing the need to assay PRL and TSH in patients with galactorrhea. These patients will respond to levothyroxine.

TSH causes not only prompt release of thyroxine hormone but also iodide transport, protein synthesis and glycosylation. The protein synthesis includes both thyroglobulin and perioxidase enzyme. TSH can increase the size of the thyroid gland by hypertrophy and hyperplasia of cells and increase vascularization.

Thyroid hormones are carried by three proteins: 1) thyroxine binding globulin (TBG), 2) thyroxine binding prealbumin, and 3) albumin. The binding to TBG is 75% to 80%. TBG may be decreased with severe liver disease and malnutrition, while estrogens increase TBG. It is best clinically to measure only TSH and free T4. With these two measurements, almost all ailments related to the thyroid dysfunction can be elucidated. TBG should not be measured routinely because there are many conditions which can cause TBG levels to vary.

Hypothyroidism

The causes of hypothyroidism in this country are usually related to antithyroid antibodies. Previously, iodine deficiency was the most important cause. Nowadays, with better nutrition, this has been eradicated. Unfortunately, hypothyroidism caused by iodine deficiency still exists in other parts of the world. Other causes include previous radioactive iodine therapy or surgery.

Symptoms of the condition include bloating, muscle cramps, weight gain, constipation, dry skin, coarse hair and irregular menstruation. Other problems can also exist, such as loss of hair from lateral areas of the eyebrows, alopecia, hypercholesterolemia, carpal tunnel syndrome, peripheral neuropathies and myxedema. In many cases, though, an astute clinician picks up a mild form of hypothyroidism, termed subclinical hypothyroidism. In this condition, the free T4 is in the normal range and the TSH is elevated. Considerable controversy exists as to whether this should be treated at all. It is best to give a trial treatment to those patients whose symptoms are significant and where the medication can be well tolerated. Treatment with levothyroxine can improve the HDL/LDL ratio.

Hyperthyroidism

The patient with hyperthyroidism can present with complaints of nervousness, heat intolerance, weight loss, sweating, palpitations and diarrhea. The critical findings can include tachycardia, warm, moist skin and proptosis. More commonly, the diagnosis is made on subtle grounds. This is confirmed with elevated free T4 and in some cases T3 levels. The TSH is very low. The causes of hyperthyroidism are toxic diffuse goiter, or Graves' disease, and toxic nodular goiter, or Plummer's disease. Exophthalmos and pretibial myxedema can be considered in the diagnosis. Graves' disease is five times more common in women than in men and could involve a circulating immune globulin. The treatment can include radioactive iodine or surgery. In women of childbearing age, propylthiouracil (PTU) is used more often.

DHEA

Dehydroepiandrosterone (DHEA) supplementation has become popular over the last few years. It should be noted that the research on this is preliminary, and the efficacy of this product is unknown at this time. There could be potential adverse effects with this product, especially if it is taken at very high doses. DHEA usage has not been well regulated. It should be noted that the adrenal gland has diminishing function as one ages. DHEA is a product of the adrenal cortex, and DHEA production is negligible by 70 years of age. In animal studies DHEA prevents obesity,[62] noninsulin diabetes[63] and tumor development.[64] It can improve cognitive tasks[65] and can reduce accelerated atherosclerosis in rabbits.[66] It can also enhance lymphocyte function and can increase interleukin-2 production.[67]

New prospective randomized studies will show whether DHEA is beneficial in human subjects. Some studies have noted a 50% reduction in heart disease with increased DHEA levels.[68] Other studies have shown mixed results in reference to (DHEA) its protective effect on the cardiovascular system.[69,70] It is clear that DHEA has a role in enhancing immune functions through increased natural killer cell activity and increased levels of interleukin-2.[71]

The adverse effects of DHEA could include liver toxicity. It may worsen the lipid profile, as there is biotransformation to testosterone. This certainly may be a factor if DHEA is given at high levels. The clinician should be aware that there may be many patients taking DHEA without a prescription and are unmonitored. At this time, DHEA cannot be recommended for menopausal or older patients. An adequate dosage of DHEA has not been established. Further studies are needed to establish efficacious dosages.[72]

MELATONIN

Melatonin is highest in childhood and adolescence; thereafter, melatonin levels decline as age progresses. Melatonin induces sleepiness, rapid-eye-movement sleep, and is thought to ameliorate jet lag. Large amounts can produce headaches and abdominal cramps. Melatonin levels are low in depressed individuals. On occasion it has been found to cause a sensation of well-being and elation. Despite the lack of adequate randomized prospective trials, melatonin is found in health food stores and is readily available to the consumer for use for its positive effects. The efficacy of this medication in old age and menopause is uncertain and it cannot be recommended at this time until further studies are reviewed.

SUMMARY

Menopause is an endocrinopathy that results from failure of the ovary, an endocrine organ; and the administration of ovarian steroids usually corrects the condition. It affects many areas of the body. Primarily these include the bone, the cardiovascular system, female genitalia and reproductive tract; new studies show that it is also implicated in cognition and memory. The lack of estrogen may contribute to Alzheimer's disease since estrogen replacement therapy decreases its risk of occurrence.[73] Estrogens have also been shown to have an antioxidant effect.[74] The use of estrogens has also been shown to prevent colon cancer.[75,76] Estrogen replacement therapy is beneficial in many circumstances.

The menopause is no longer a short-lived state, as it was in earlier centuries. We are learning a great deal about how this estrogen-deprived state can affect women. Future studies could show that DHEA may be used to improve immune function in menopause and old age, and that melatonin usage may improve sleep-related problems in menopause and old age.

REFERENCES

1 Kannel WB: Metabolic risk factors for coronary heart disease in women: Prospective from the Farmingham study. *Am Heart J* 1987; 114: 413.

2 Ravnikar VA: Compliance with hormone replacement therapy. Are women receiving the full impact of hormone replacement therapy preventative health benefits? *Women's Health Issues* 1992; 2: 75–82.

3 Baker TG, Sum OW: Development of the ovary and oogenesis. *Clin Obstet Gynecol* 1976; 3–26.

4 Hughes FM Jr, Gorospe WC: Biochemical identification of apoptosis (Programmed). In granulosa cells: Evidence for a potential mechanism underlying follicular atresia. *Endocrinology* 1991; 129: 2415–2422.

5 Thomford PJ, Jelovsek FR, Mattison DR: Effect of oocyte number and rate of atregia on the age of menopause. *Reprod Toxicol* 1987; 1: 41–51.

6 Regulation of the Menstrual Cycle, In: Speroff L, Glass RH, Kase NG eds.: *Clinical Gynecologic Endocrinology and Infertility*, 5th edn., Williams and Wilkins, 1994; 183–233.

7 Rivier C, Rivier J, Vale W: Inhibin-mediated feedback control of follicle stimulating hormone secretion in the female rat. *Science* 1986; 234: 205.

8 Vicsak TA, Tucker EM, Cappel S, et al.: Hormonal regulation of granulosa cell inhibin diosynthesis. *Endocrinology* 1986; 119: 2711.

9 Lenton EA, DeKretser DN, Woodward AJ, Robertston DM: Inhibin concentrations throughout the menstrual cycles of normal, infertile, and older women compared with those during spontaneous conception cycles. *J Clin Endo Metab* 1991; 73: 1180.

10 Ling N, Ying S, Ueno N, et al.: Pituitary FSH is released by a heterodimer of the beta subunits from the two forms of hemadin. *Nature* 1986; 321: 779.

11 Buckler HM, Evans A, Mamlora H, Burger HG, Anderson DC: Gonadotropin, steroid and inhibin levels in women with incipient ovarian failure during anovulatory and ovulatory rebound cycles. *J Clin Endo Metab* 1991; 72: 116.

12 Speroff L, Glass RH, Kase NE: Menopause and postmenopausal hormonal therapy. In: *Clinical Gynecological Endocrinology and Infertility*, 5th edn. Baltimore, MD: Williams and Wilkins, 1994; 583–650.

13 Goswamy RK, Campbell S, Royston JP, et al. Ovarian size in postmenopausal woman. *Br J Obstet Gynecol* 1988; 75: 795.

14 Longcope C, Hunter R, Franz C: Steroid secretion by the postmenopausal ovary. *Am J Obstet Gynecol* 1980; 138: 564.

15 Mattingly RF, Huang WY: Steroidogenesis of the menopausal ovary. *J Obstet Gynecol* 1969; 62: 508.

16 Duponte Labrie F, Luu-Thev Pellipier G: Immunocyto chemical localization of three beta-hydroxysteroid dehydrogenase-delta 5-delta 4-isomerase in human ovary. *J Clin Endo Metab* 1992; 74: 994.

17 Dennefors BL, Janson PO, Hamberger L, Knutson F: Hilus cells from human postmenopausal ovaries: Sensitivity, steroid and cyclic-amp production. *Acta Obstet Gynecol Scand* 1982; 61: 413.

18 Greenblatt RB, Colle ML, Mahesh VP: Ovarian and adrenal steroid production in the postmenopausal ovary. *Obstet Gynecol* 1976; 47: 383.

19 Braithwaite SS, Erkman–Balis B, Avila TD: Postmenopausal virilization due to ovarian stromal hypothecosis. *J Clin Endo Metab* 1978; 46: 295–300.

20 Van-Heyningen C, MacFarlane IA, Diver MJ, Muronda C, Tuffnell D: Virilization due to ovarian hyperthecosis in a postmenopausal woman. *Gynecol Endo* 1988; 2: 331–338.

21 Goldman JM, Kapadia JL: Virilization in a postmenopausal woman due to ovarian stromal hyperthecosis. *Postgrad Med J* 1991; 67: 304–306.

22 Leedman BJ, Bierre AR, Martin FIR: Virilizing nodular stromal hyperthecosis, diabetes mellitus, and insulin resistance in the postmenopausal woman. Case report. *Br J Obstet Gynecol* 1989; 96: 1095–1098.

23 Adashi EY: The climacteric ovary. A viable endocrine organ. *Seminars in Reprod Endo* 1991; 9: 200.

24 Adashi EY: The climacteric ovary. In: Adashi EY, Rock JA, Rosenwaks Z, eds. *Reproductive Endocrinology, Surgery and Technology*. vol. 2, Philadelphia, PA: Lippincott-Raven, 1996; 1745–1757.

25 Judd HL, Lucas WE, Yen SSC: Effect of oophorectomy on circulating testosterone and androstenedione levels in patients with endometrial cancer. *Am J Obstet Gynecol* 1974; 118: 739.

26 Peluso JJ, Steger RW, Jaszczak S, Hafez ESE: Gonadotropin binding sites in human postmenopausal ovaries. *Fertil Steril* 1976; 27: 789.

27 Nakano R, Shima K, Yamoto M, Kobayashi M, Nishimori K, Hiraoka J: Binding sites for gonadotropins in human postmenopausal ovaries. *Obstet Gynecol* 1989; 73: 196.

28 Poliaka Jones GES, Goldberg B, Solomon D, Woodruff ID: Effect of human chorionic gonadotropin on postmenopausal woman. *Am J Obstet Gynecol* 1968; 101: 731.

29 Rabinovici J, Rothman P, Monroe SE, Nerenberg C, Jaffe RB: Endocrine effects and pharmacokinetic characteristics of a potent new gonadotropin-releasing hormone antagonist (Ganirelix) with minimal histamine releasing properties. Studies in Postmenopausal Women. *J Clin Endo Metab* 1992; 75: 1220.

30 Hagsta TA, Janson PO: The epidemiology of climacteric symptoms. *Acta Obset Gynecol Scand* 1986; 134(supp): 59.

31 Erlik Y, Pataryn IV, Muldrum DR, *et al*.: Association of awaking episodes with menopausal hot flashes. *JAMA* 1981; 245: 741.

32 Grodin JM, Siiteri PK, McDonald PC: Source of estrogen production in postmenopausal women. *J Clin Endo Metab* 1973; 36: 207.

33 Davidson DJ, Gambone JC, Lagasse LD, *et al*.: Free estradiol in postmenopausal women with and without endometrial cancer. *J Clini Endo Metab* 1981; 52: 404.

34 Walsh BW, Schiff I: The hot flash: Impact of sex steroid replacement. In: *Reproductive Endocrinology Surgery and Technology*. Adashi EY, Rock JA, Rosenwaks Z, eds. Philadelphia, PA: Lippincott Raven, 1996; 1841–1850.

35 Beattie CW, Rodgers CH, Soyka LF: Influence of ovariectomy and ovarian steroids on hypothalamic pyricine hydroxylase activity in the rat. *Endo* 1972; 91: 276.

36 Luine BN, McEwen BS: Effect of estradiol on tyrosine hydroxylase of Type A monomine oxidase in brain. *J Neuro Chem* 1977; 28: 1221.

37 Nixon RL, Jamowski DS, Davis JM: Effects of progesterone, estradiol and testosterone on the uptake and metabolism of ^{3}H–norepinephrine, ^{3}H-dopamine, and ^{3}H-seratonin in rat synatosones. *Res Commun Chem Pathol Pharmacol* 1974; 7: 233.

38 Johnson AE, Nock B, McEwen B, *et al*.: Estradiol modulation of noradronergic receptors in the guinea pig brain assessed by tritium-sensitive film audoradiography. *Brain Res* 1985; 336: 153.

39 Clayden JR, Bell JW, Pollard P: Menopausal flushing: Double blind trial of nonhormonal medication. *Br Med J* 1974; 1: 49.

40 Edington RF, Chagnon JP, Steinberg WN: Clonidine for menopausal flushing. *Can Med Assoc J* 1980; 123: 23.

41 Freedman RR, Woodward S, Sabharwal SC: Alpha$_2$ adrenergic mechanism in menopausal hot-flushes. *Obstet Gynecol* 1990; 76: 573.

42 Lindsay R: The burden of osteoporosis: Cost. *Am J Med* 1995; 98: S9–11.

43 Melton LJ III, Lane AW, Cooper C, Eastell R, O'Fallon WN, Riggs BL: Prevalence and incidence of vertigo deformities. *Osteo Int* 1993; 3: 113–119.

44 Christiansen C: Menopausal osteoporosis: Impact of sex steroid replacement. In: *Reproductive Endocrinology, Surgery and Technology*, vol. 2, Adashi EY, Rock JA, Rosenwaks Z, eds. Philadelphia, PA: Lippincott Raven, 1996; 1825–1839.

45 Whitteman JCM, Grobbee DE, Kok FJ, Hofman A, Valkenburg HA: Increased risk of atherosclerosis in women after the menopause. *Br Med J* 1989; 298: 642–644.

46 *Advanced Report of Final Monthly Statistics*. 1989 Monthly Vital Statistics REP, 1992; 40(supp 2): 1247.

47 Miller VT, Muesing RA, LaRosa JC, *et al*.: Effects of conjugated equine estrogen with and without three different progestogens and lipoproteins. High density lipoprotein subfractions and apolipoprotein-1. *Obstet Gynecol* 1991; 77: 235–240.

48 Sullivan JM, Zwaag RE, Lemp GF, *et al*.: Postmenopausal estrogen use and coronary atherosclerosis. *Anals Int Med* 1988; 108: 358–363.

49 Williams JK, Shively CA, Clarkson TB: Determinants of coronary artery reactivity in premenopausal female synomolgous monkeys and diet-induced atherosclerosis. *Circulation* 1994; 90: 983–987.

50 Reis SE, Gloth SG, Blumenthal RS, *et al*.: Ethinyl estradiol acutely attenuates abnormal coronary vasomotor responses to acetylcholine in postmenopausal women. *Circulation* 1994; 89: 52–60.

51 Rosano GMC, *et al*.: Estrogen improves exercise-induced myocardial ischemia in female patients with coronary artery disease. *Lancet* 1993; 342: 133–136.

52 VanBuren GA, Yang D, Clark KE: Estrogen-induced uterine vasodilation is antagonized by L-metroarginine methylester, an inhibitor of nitric oxide synthesis. *Am J Obstet Gynecol* 1992; 167: 828–833.

53 Wild RA: Estrogen: Effects on the cardiovascular tree. *Obstet Gynecol* 1996; 87(2)(supp): 27–35.

54 Lasordo DW, Kearney M, Kim EA, Jekanowski J, Isner JM: Variable expression of the estrogen receptor in normal and atherosclerotic coronary arteries of premenopausal woman. *Circulation* 1994; 89: 1501–1510.

55 Sarrel PM, Lufkin EG, Oursler MJ, Keefe D: Estrogen actions in arteries, bones, and brain. *Sci Am Science Med* 1994; 1: 44–53.

56 Hammond CB: Menopause and hormone replacement therapy; An overview. *Obstet Gynecol* 1996; 87(2)(supp): 2–15.

57 Bachman GA, Lieblum SR, Grill J: Brief sexual inquiry in a gynecologic practice. *Obstet Gynecol* 1989; 73: 425–427.

58 Bhatia NN, Bergman A, Karram MM: Effects of estrogen on urethral function in women with urinary incontinence. *Am J Obstet Gynecol* 1989; 160: 176–181.

59 Wilson PD, Faragher B, Butler B, *et al*.: Treatment with all piperazine oestrone sulfate for general stress urinary incontinence in postmenopausal women. *Br J Obstet Gynaecol* 1989; 394: 568.

60 McEwen BS: The brain as a target organ of endocrine hormones. In: Kreiger DT, Hughes JS, eds. *Neuroendocrinology*. Sunderland: Sinauer Associates, 1980.

61 Luine VN, McEwen BS: Effect of estradiol on turnover of Type A monomine oxidase in brain. *J Neurochem* 1977; 28: 1221–1227.

62 Yen TT, Allan JV, Pearson DB: Prevention of obesity in AVY/A mice by dehydroepiandrosterone. *Lipids* 1977; 12: 409.

63 Coleman OL, Leiter EH, Schwizer RW: Therapeutic effects of dehydroepiandrosterone (DHEA) in diabetic mice. *Diabetes* 1982; 31: 830.

64 Schwartz AG, Pashko LL: Cancer chemoprevention with the adrenocorticosteroid dehydroepiandrosterone and structural analogs. *J Cell Biochem* 1993; 17G: 73.

65 Roberts E: Dehydroepiandrosterone (DHEA) and its sulfate (DHEAS) has no facilitators (effects on the brain tissue in culture and on memory in young and old mice. A cyclic GNP hypothesis of action of DHEA and DHEAS in nervous system and other tissues). In: Kalimi M, Regelson W, eds. *The Biologic Role of Dehydroepiandrosterone (DHEA)*. Berlin: Walter DE Gruyder, 1990; 1342.

66 Eich DM, Nestler JE, Johnson DE, *et al.*: Inhibition of accelerated coronary atherosclerosis with dehydroepiandrosterone in the heterotopic rabbit model of cardiac transplantation. *Circulation* 1993; 87: 261.

67 Daynes RA, Dudley DJ, Araneo BA: Regulation of new lymphokine production in vivo (dehydroepiandrosterone is a natural enhancer of interleukin-2 synthesis by helper T-cells). *European J Immunol* 1990; 20: 793.

68 Barrett-Connor E, Khaw KT, Yen SSC: A prospective study of dehydroepiandrosterone sulfate, mortality and cardiovascular disease. *N Eng J Med* 1986; 315: 1519.

69 Barrett-Connor E, Goodman-Gruen D: Dehydroepiandrosterone sulfate does not predict cardiovascular death in postmenopausal women. *Circulation* 1995; 91: 1757.

70 Barrett-Connor E, Goodman-Gruen D: The epidemiology of DHEAS and cardiovascular disease. In: Beloino FL, Daynes RA, Hornsby PJ, *et al.*, eds. *Dehydroepiandrosterone and Aging*. 77, 4th ed. New York Academy of Science, 1995; 259–270.

71 Casson PR, Andersen RN, Herrod HG, *et al.*: Oral dehydroepiandrosterone in physiologic doses modulates immune function in postmenopausal women. *Am J Obstet Gynecol* 1993; 169: 1536–1539.

72 Casson PR, Buster JE: DHEA replacement after menopause: HRT 2000 or nostrum of the 90's? *Contemp Ob/Gyn* 1997; 42(4): 119.

73 Sherman BB, Harper D: Estrogen and memory in postmenopausal women without Alzheimer's disease. Presented at the Third Annual Meeting of the North American Menopause Society, Cleveland OH, September 17, 1992.

74 Wilcox JC, Hwang J, Hodis HN, Sevanian A, Stanczyk FZ, Lobo RA: Cardioprotective effects of individual conjugated equine estrogens through their possible modulation of insulin resistance and oxidation of low density lipoprotein. *Fertil Steril* 1997; 67(1): 57–62.

75 Newcomb PA, Storer BE: Postmenopausal hormone use and risk of large bowel cancer. *J Nat Cancer Inst* 1995; 87(14): 1039–1040,1067–1071.

76 Calle EE, Miracle-McMahill HL, Thrin ML, Health CW Jr.: Estrogen replacement therapy and risk of fatal colon cancer in a prospective cohort of postmenopausal women. *J Nat Cancer Inst* 1995; 87(7): 517–523.

3

Emotional aspects of the perimenopause

MICHAL ARTAL

The perimenopause and the menopause which follows are both biological phenomena correlating with hormonal events.

The strict meaning of the word menopause is the woman's last menstrual period. Both the medical literature and the lay public use the term menopause more broadly, as the period of time following the last menstrual cycle.[1,2,3]

Other common nonmedical names used are: the change; change of life; the transition; climacteric. The word 'climacter' originates from the Greek *klimakter*: a step of a ladder. Long before the discovery of ovarian hormones, climacter originally referred to the stage of midlife for both men and women. Over time, though, climacter has been used to refer to the female midlife.

HISTORICAL OVERVIEW

It is fascinating to follow a myth longitudinally over centuries to see how it originates and how it is cultivated, maintained and promulgated. Through the story of Sarah's giving birth to Isaac, the Old Testament tells of attitudes of disbelief and ridicule at the idea of sexuality and conception in the postmenopause. The word 'Isaac' in Hebrew literally means 'will laugh' (Genesis 18: 11–12).

Historically, Western culture associated the menopause with significant disturbances of mood and behavior.[4,5] Medical writers implicated menopause with manifestations ranging from neurasthenia-like disorders[6] to 'pain, giddiness of the head, hysteric disorders, colic pains and female weakness' . . . often very troublesome to others.[7] The same eighteenth century medical text blamed the cause of such menopausal disturbances on 'the many excesses introduced by luxury and the irregularities of the passion'.[7] An early 1850s gynecological text[8] states in a chapter on the change of life: 'The sense of melancholy, decadence of the constitution . . . an old woman with gradual decay of physical attraction.'

Attitudes and expectations affect all members of society – men and women as well as physicians. Similar negative views of menopause and of women at midlife could be found in the nonmedical literature as well. Seventeenth to twentieth century literature depicted middle-aged women as irrational and unnaturally sexual. Shakespeare's *Hamlet* expresses these prevailing societal attitudes that sexuality in middle-aged women is unnatural when he protested his mother's behavior: 'You cannot call it love, for at our age the heyday in the blood is tame, it's humble.'[9]

Menopause and postmenopausal women were consistently portrayed in myth and folklore as angry, meddlesome, irritable, malevolent, physically unappealing, frequently generating fear, disgust and ridicule. Many fairy tales conjure up stereotypical images of middle-aged women as witches and wicked stepmothers.

An early 1920s gynecological text states: 'The majority of women in the menopause have psychic symptoms . . . They are peevish, irritable, morose and depressed . . . The various psychoses of the menopause constitute an important group . . . Many have full blown insanity with melancholia, paranoia and maniacal conditions.'[11] Some writers formalized menopausal disturbances by creating the diagnosis of involutional melancholia.[10,11]

The concept of this agitated depression as a specific involutional clinical syndrome was later discarded and relegated to psychiatric history.[12,13] It was finally removed from the third edition of the *Diagnostic and Statistical Manual* in 1980.

Increasingly more refined epidemiological research over the past 25 years has consistently found no evidence for a specific depressive syndrome occurring during the perimenopause or menopausal years.[14,15] Studies that have analyzed age-specific risks for mood disorders in the perimenopause found no increase in the total or in new episodes of depression during this phase of life.[16–19] Likewise, large-scale epidemiological studies have failed to find an increase in depression in menopausal women compared with other periods of female life.[20–25]

In summary, recent data consistently show that major depression is not more prevalent during perimenopause and menopause, and that most women do not experience severe depression during this period. Yet some women do report distressing symptoms of irritability, tearfulness, insomnia, fatigue and decreased memory and concentration during the perimenopause.[26–28] How can we account for these perimenopausal complaints? Can the perspective of 'some grain of truth' be helpful to shed some light on these findings?

In nonpsychiatric medical literature, one frequently finds that no differentiation is made between depressive symptoms, transient depressed mood and depressive syndrome.[29] The terms depressive symptoms, sadness, tearful mood, negative mood, depression, depression scores on self-rating questionnaires, mood dysfunction, psychological dysfunction, low affect, the blues, low mood and dysphoric mood are frequently used interchangeably, and are considered as equivalents of clinical depression. Clarification of the terms might be helpful.

Mood is the internal/subjective experience of one's feelings. *Affect* is the behavioral expression of the mood.

The qualities of both can be mild and transient or pervasive and long-standing. The diagnosis of clinical depression can be made only if the duration and intensity meet specific criteria.[30] A sad mood may be a normal reaction to a wide variety of disappointments or losses including health problems. It is not to be confused with depression.

One of the most vexing difficulties of depression research in the menopause is how to interpret the relationship between hormonal events and emotional/behavioral phenomena.

Hormonal changes do not occur in isolation, and other stressors invariably impinge upon menopausal women: aging, the prospect of declining health and the growing awareness of mortality. How do we account for the respective contributions of these variables, and what is the nature of their interactions?

While the hormonal changes and the cessation of menses are the biological markers of perimenopause and menopause, a multitude of other symptoms has been reported by some women. These include hot flashes, sleep disturbances, apprehension, irritability, decreased concentration and decreased or loss of sexual desire. The incidence of these symptoms varies in different populations.[2,3] These adverse symptoms have long been associated with menopause. The nature of their association has come under increased scrutiny, with three main explanations offered.[29]

1 *The estrogen deficiency theory*: The association is biological and causal. Some even claim that these symptoms are specific to the menopause.
2 *The domino effect theory*: The association between negative symptoms and estrogen decline is not causal but, rather, indirect. The estrogen decline causes hypoestrogenic somatic symptoms (vasomotor symptoms and urogenital atrophy), and it is their effect that causes negative emotional reactions.
3 *The psychosocial theory*: Depression, if present, is only coincidental to the endocrine changes. It is the outcome of other, nonhormonal events that women may experience at this time of their lives.

I will review the most relevant research literature and data encompassing these three perspectives.

1. The estrogen deficiency theory

The approach of estrogen deficiency theory related research has been to focus exclusively on biological variables. The biological variable most frequently used has been the level of circulating ovarian hormones. This was then assumed to produce the emotional/behavioral data of the sample groups of perimenopausal or menopausal women attending menopause clinics.

A primary causal association has been proposed between declining levels of circulating estrogen and negative moods.[31] Specific intracellular estrogen and testosterone receptors have been identified in several brain regions.[32] This may be a mechanism by which the sex hormones influence mood, cognition, behavior and sexuality.

Potential pathophysiological mechanisms implicated are as follows. Estrogen has stimulatory effects on several brain mechanisms:

- Estrogen increases the rate of degradation of monoamine oxidase (MAO), the enzyme that catabolizes the neurotransmitter serotonin.[33] This increases serotonin bioavailability.
- Estrogen displaces tryptophan, the precursor of serotonin, from its binding sites to plasma albumin,[34] thereby allowing more free tryptophan to be available to the brain, where it is metabolized to serotonin.

According to the biogenic amine hypothesis of depression, a decrease in brain serotonin levels may play a role in depression.[35] Since estrogen increases bioavailability of serotonin, a decrease of circulating estrogen is implicated in negative moods.

- Estrogen lowers the brain seizure threshold. The relevance of this action to mood is unclear. A possible mechanism might be the enhancing of interneuronal transmission.

- Of potential importance to memory functions is the enzyme choline acetyltransferase (CAT), which is needed for acetylcholine synthesis.[36] A decrease in brain concentration of acetylcholine was reported in Alzheimer's disease.[37] Estrogen may enhance memory by increasing the activity of CAT.[36,41]
- Progesterone has the opposite effects both on MAO and on dopamine. The net effect is the lowering of brain levels of serotonin, which may play a role in lowering mood.
- Progesterone increases brain seizure threshold and lowers brain excitability.[31,38–40] Clinically, progesterone induces somnolence.

The salient findings of the research data looking at the possible association between mood and ovarian hormones can be divided into two distinct groups:

1 Studies on clinically depressed menopausal women.
2 Studies on nondepressed menopausal women.

There have been three published reports on the effects of exogenous estrogen on clinically depressed menopausal women: Kleiber and colleagues[42] claimed successful results; their results have not been replicated. Two later studies, by Schneider and colleagues and by Oppenheim and colleagues found that giving estrogen to clinically depressed menopausal women failed to improve their depression.[43,44] Schneider further cautions against making the assumption that psychological changes during menopause are caused by hormonal changes: 'One of the negative consequences of this assumption is the view that the emotional problems can be remedied by hormone replacement alone, with resultant failure to investigate other possible factors.'[43]

Another approach was taken by Sherwin, who looked at nondepressed women before and after surgical menopause.[45,46] The cohort was divided into four groups: women receiving estrogen replacement, androgen replacement, combined estrogen and androgen replacement, and placebo only.

Looking at the results, it is evident that none of the oophorectomized women in the placebo group (who received no HRT) developed clinical depression. This is an important finding that was not emphasized by the author. Even the abrupt fall in ovarian hormones did not cause clinical depression in any of the women in the study. Since none of the women were depressed either before or following the surgical menopause, Sherwin looked at their relative scores on the Beck Depression Inventory (BDI). Their scores on the BDI were higher than hormone-treated women but never reached the threshold level of clinical depression. The BDI scores of the hormone-treated women were lower, again not reaching the depression threshold.

Sherwin conducted several studies looking at the nature of the association between mood and ovarian hormones. Her studies were blinded, and levels of circulating ovarian hormone were measured. All her study patients were a special group. All were women attending a menopause clinic, rather than menopausal women in the nonclinical population. This is already a selective group of patients. Extrapolating data to all menopausal women, including menopausal women without complaints, is questionable.

All Sherwin's studies, with the exception of one[47] were done on a cohort of surgically menopausal women. Again, caution must be exercised before extrapolating data from surgical menopause to natural menopause. All the studies were carried out on nondepressed women.

Three qualifying observations have to be made:

- While the studies are taken to prove a primary mood-elevating effect of estrogen, one cannot exclude the possibility that the mood improvement may have resulted from the correction of vasomotor and other somatic hypoestrogenic symptoms in the group receiving HRT.

• Regardless whether estrogen mood-enhancing actions are primary, secondary or a combination of both, estrogen effects do not appear to have a therapeutic utility for clinically depressed menopausal women. Elevating mood scores on a BDI questionnaire in nondepressed patients and alleviating depression in clinically depressed patients are two different things.

• The design of all the endocrine studies so far has focused exclusively on hormonal variables only, to the exclusion of any psychosocial variable. If questions are not being asked, other variables are not looked at nor evaluated – potentially important information is not likely to be found. If we do not look for something, we are not likely to find it. The results of such research might be misleading in the sense that they are overly reductionistic.

2. The domino effect theory

Rather than a primary causal association between declining estrogen levels and negative moods, a domino effect is proposed. Declining estrogen levels cause somatic hypoestrogenic symptoms. These somatic symptoms may be sufficiently disruptive to cause the psychological manifestations experienced by some perimenopausal women.[25,29,48,49]

Hot flashes are the most frequently reported symptom of the perimenopause, experienced by 60%[3] to 75% to 85%[2] of all women undergoing natural menopause, and frequently also reported as the most disruptive symptom. The onset of the flash is unpredictable. It may be accompanied by a headache, palpitations, profuse perspiration and chills. It is frequently reported as a source of embarrassment and disruption in social and in work situations. When occurring at night, the hot flashes disrupt sleep (night sweats) causing insomnia and sleep deprivations.[50] Like a domino effect, the insomnia leads to sleep deprivation, fatigue, nervousness, irritability and resultant impaired concentration.

Vaginal atrophic changes contribute to dyspareunia. Urinary frequency and pelvic floor relaxation are likely to interfere with daily life. These disruptive somatic symptoms can become an important cause of impairment of women's quality of life during the perimenopause. According to this theory, when negative moods and apprehension are present, they should be understood as a reaction to the cascading interference in women's lives. Indeed, an increase in the frequency of office visits and of complaints of both physical and emotional distress are reported during the perimenopause.[2,51]

Not until 1975 was the study of the pathophysiology of hot flashes systematically undertaken.[52] In the past, women were frequently told it was all in their heads. Menopausal women were frequently prescribed sedatives and tranquilizers such as bromides, phenobarbital, librium and valium. Not infrequently this resulted in prescription drug dependency. This practice still persists in many circles, with Prozac and other antidepressants being frequently prescribed to women.

The somatic symptoms readily respond to estrogen replacement which frequently alleviates the apprehension and the other psychological reactions.[25,48,49] Campbell and Whitehead[43] concluded that estrogen exerted its benefit by alleviating the somatic symptoms.[49] In their study, the psychological symptoms of women who did not have hot flashes at the outset showed no benefit in their psychological symptoms from the estrogen. It is not surprising that disruptive somatic symptoms, to the extent that they diminish quality of life, will affect mood. These negative symptoms ought not to be confused with clinical depression, however. Emotional distress is not depression. If a perimenopausal woman is severely depressed, one has to look for another etiology and for another form of treatment. Estrogen given to severely depressed menopausal women failed to alleviate their depression.[43,44]

3. The psychosocial theory

Most women do not experience depression during this period of their lives. A first episode of depression without a prior history may be due to psychosocial stressors that are common to this stage of life.[53–55] An extensive literature has emerged that looks at the stressors of midlife.[56–58] The main life events and consequent psychological stressors of midlife are:

1 Undeniable signs of aging.
2 Increasing likelihood of illness in oneself or spouse.
3 Children move away from home and establish their own families.
4 Illness of parents, caring for ailing parents and death of parents.
5 Increasing awareness of the finiteness of life.
6 Realization that not all of one's goals can be fulfilled; realization of lost time and lost opportunities.

These experiences are similar for both genders and frequently contribute to what has been referred to as 'midlife crisis'. Its hallmark is one's responses to the taking stock, the uncertainty about the future and one's awareness of the finite nature of time and of life. While these midlife experiences in women coincide chronologically with menopause, they are not causally related to its hormonal changes.[53,59,64]

About life events it is important to keep in mind that it is not life events themselves but, rather, their meanings for the individual person which will determine their emotional impact. This presents a special complexity for psychiatric research: it is easier to identify and document events; it is more difficult to ascertain their meanings and therefore their emotional impact for a given patient. Eisenberg reminds us that: 'In clinical practice it is the particularities and the idiosyncrasies of the individual patient that challenge the physician . . . and that medicine includes but cannot be reduced to molecular biology.'[62] Similar ideas have been expressed by George Engel when he formulated the biopsychosocial model of medicine.[63]

While midlife stresses are similar for both genders, women may have greater vulner-abilities.[60,61] As a group, many women have been and are still expected to have a greater involvement with parenting than with career, as compared to men. Women whose identities have been closely tied to their mothering role may experience distress when children leave home.[61] Because of the common experience of many women to feel conflicted around their mothering role versus their career, women are more vulnerable to feel guilt and self-blame if the departing child experiences difficulties.

The empty-nest syndrome illustrates how the same life experience may have very different personal meaning and therefore different emotional impact on different individuals. For the woman who has centred her life around her children and her maternal role, children leaving home may stir feelings of loss, depression and a sense that her useful life may be over. For another it may mean new freedom and being restored to herself and to her own development.[61,65] Margot Tallmer in 'Empty-Nest Syndrome: Possibility or Despair,' challenges the common view that women predominantly experience menopause and children leaving home as losses. Emotional distress may in fact result from the return of adult children when the menopausal woman is eager to relinquish the care-taking role.[65]

Because of prevailing cultural idealization of feminine youthful physique, women as a group tend to be more preoccupied than men with their physical attractiveness and may be more vulnerable to negative feelings when physical signs of aging appear. The common expression 'older women look older, while older men look more distinguished' illustrates this attitude.

As a group women tend to live longer than men and also tend to have a lower income and are less financially secure. Fears of being alone, of illness, of helplessness and of poverty are therefore more common in women.[18,26,53]

SOCIOECONOMIC STATUS

Another nonhormonal variable linked to emotional distress at the menopause is women's socioeconomic status. Studies show that, while vasomotor symptoms directly attributable to hypoestrogenism have similar prevalence across socioeconomic and demographic groups, psychological distress and related negative symptoms were higher among women of lower socioeconomic status compared to women of higher socioeconomic class.[26,27,66,67] Women of the first group have low income, frequently lower educational level, and limited employment satisfaction, and show higher prevalence of negative symptoms during menopause.[68] Since these women as a group are more likely to have more psychosocial stressors (financial problems, less life satisfaction, lower self-esteem), yet are not distinct endocrinologically, a likely conclusion from these studies is the causal importance of nonhormonal factors to mood.

Manifestations of menopause in heterogeneous sociocultural groups may help differentiate physiological from cultural variables. If menopausal symptoms result principally from hormonal events, one would expect women throughout the world to experience similar symptoms.[73]

Cross-cultural studies show that the prevalence of negative symptoms, both vasomotor and other somatic and negative symptoms, vary significantly across different cultures.[69,70,72,73] In Western cultures, hot flashes are the only symptom systematically associated with the menopause.[22,26] Several studies show very few or a lack of negative symptoms in those societies where women have a respected and valued role after the menopause, or where they enjoy relatively greater freedom compared to their earlier life when they had been restricted by taboos, had to be veiled and frequently were believed to be contaminated by menstrual blood.[71-73]

In conclusion, all the above studies seem to suggest the importance of psychosocial factors to the clinical and behavioral manifestations of the menopause.

SEXUALITY AND MENOPAUSE

A decline in sexual interest and in sexual activity in menopause and postmenopause had long been a widely held belief[8,75] and sexuality in postmenopausal women was seen as an aberration. Old religious traditions limiting sexuality to reproduction might be one likely source. While women's reproductive potential ends with the ovarian senescence at menopause, men's reproductive potential continues until a much older age. Historically, some cultures sanctioned taking additional younger wives by men for purposes of producing additional offspring. No data exist documenting the emotional responses of menopausal women thus shunned by husbands and society. It is certainly logical to conclude that their sense of self-esteem and self-worth would be negatively affected if the end of their reproductive capabilities also led to their diminished status.

Reference has been made to the biblical story of elderly Sarah, who laughed at the thought of being sexual in her old age. The Bible also tells how upset she was when Abraham took another wife to bear him more children (Genesis 18: 11–12). A mid-1850s' gynecological text states: 'After all what is sex? It is reproductive power . . . In women the sex organs are different, they are subject to the tide of life.'[8] One can certainly see a logical parallel between the two historically held beliefs about menopause – that menopause was a time of a serious mental as well as sexual decline for women.

In humans, sexual desire and its expression are complex phenomena influenced by many variables, both psychological and biological. Among the psychological factors are one's individual psychology, availability and attitude of one's partner, and the contribution of prevailing sociocultural attitudes.[76] Given the historically prevailing attitude of a sexual decline in menopause, many women feel embarrassed or improper being sexual after middle age. This belief can become a self-fulfilling prophecy. More recent data have emerged reporting that women who were sexually active before menopause will have fewer problems and will continue to have satisfactory sexual activity after menopause.[77–79] Brecher published the largest and most comprehensive study of sexuality in the aging population since Kinsey in 1938.[79] His sample included 4246 men and women over the age of 50. Comparing married women with married men showed that their level of sexual activity was almost identical. Other, more recent studies report that many menopausal women become more active sexually after the fear of pregnancy is removed by menopause.[72,80]

Vaginal atrophy due to hypoestrogenism may lead to painful intercourse.[78] This and the other hypoestrogenic somatic symptoms may add to apprehension and other negative moods. Effective management includes educating the patient, recommending the use of lubricants and alleviating the hypoestrogenic symptoms by HRT.

The prescribing of testosterone to menopausal women to enhance sexual desire has been reported.[81,82] Several studies report the negative effects of MPA (medroxyprogesterone acetate) on sexual desire.[83,84] Sherwin reported that MPA dampened sexual desire in postmenopausal women receiving combined estrogen–progestin replacement in a sequential regimen.[85]

Libido may be adversely affected both by the decline in testosterone availability after menopause as well as by hormone replacement with estrogen and progesterone. The addition of systemic or topical testosterone has been shown to improve libido in menopausal and postmenopausal women.[82]

CONCLUDING REMARKS

The hormonal effects of the perimenopause and menopause are difficult to disentangle from the effects of emotionally significant midlife experiences. This difficulty may be overlooked by focusing on hormonal effects and ignoring psychosocial variables. This is tempting because it offers simplicity to practitioners and to researchers alike. It narrows the mutidimensional field to simpler medical algorithms. It reduces psychological considerations merely to background noise. It is further tempting because it allows us to seek refuge in biomedical thinking, to distance ourselves from unpleasant feelings of uncertainty, vulnerability and loss, both in our patients and in ourselves. This is true for practitioners of both genders.

A narrow focus on female hormonal changes may allow male physicians to reduce their own fears of aging, of declining memory and of the other common midlife experiences by relegating them to the hormonal menopause and therefore of no consequence to men. Data derived solely from biomedical research readily lend themselves to measurements and numerical tabulations. This offers simplicity and confers an aura of scientific objectivity.

Psychosocial events and their meanings are difficult to study. Individual differences add complexity to diagnosis, to treatment and to research.

The simplest answers, as tempting and expedient as they may be, are not necessarily the most accurate, however.

These considerations may explain the controversies in the relative contributions of endocrine versus psychosocial factors to the psychological phenomena of menopause. It is this author's opinion that these are also some of the reasons behind the recent growing focus on the biomedical model as the explanatory model for depression.

Assertions have been made that the ovarian hormones, estrogen and progesterone, are the cause of depression in women.[86,87] These assertions went even farther to invoke ovarian hormone fluctuations as the explanation for the higher prevalence of depression in women.

Three additional 'conditions' have been implicated as casualties of the normal endocrinological events of the female reproductive cycle: premenstrual syndrome, climacteric depression and postpartum depression.

This remains an unproved theory. It is also an ideology, an ideology of biological determinism of a particular kind, an old kind. According to this theory, the female sex is inherently flawed because aspects of normal female physiology (ovarian hormone cycles) are at the root cause of mental illness in women. Like any ideology, it has its own motives, beliefs and potential blind spots. The resurrection of the 'anatomy is destiny' myth seems to be one of them. This theory stigmatizes women as less stable, less reliable and at the destructive mercy of their hormones.

The effects of such an ideology are potentially staggering. Women are led to believe that their biology puts them in danger of mental illness, that their ovarian hormones are to blame for their ills. Since this theory denies that depression may have environmental causes, its proponents also tell women that they should not look at their environment for potential causes for their depression. Women should, instead, look at their ovarian hormones as the cause of their problems. According to this theory, women's ovaries are the root cause of the excess depression in women.

The published finding that surgical menopause failed to precipitate depression in women who were not receiving HRT[45,46] seems to contradict the assertion that falling levels of ovarian hormones are sufficient cause for depression. Curiously, this received little or no attention.

Another, often-forgotten, simple fact remains that the large majority of women menstruate, give birth and undergo menopause without becoming emotionally ill, irrational or depressed. There are millions and millions of such reproductive events and, lest we forget, they are normal physiological processes.

Losses, disappointments and low self-esteem do play an important etiological role in many depressions. Environmental factors surely may precipitate such emotions. While brain chemistry affects emotions, it is important to remember that emotions affect brain chemistry. Sex hormones also affect the brain. These are well-known facts, and any responsible research must consider their interactions and respective contributions. Looking at patients with this perspective in mind, rather than a simplistic either/or attitude, will serve the practitioner well and will do right by the patient. Patients are more than the collective of their molecules. Illness and its manifestations in a given patient are influenced by a lifetime of individual experience.

When faced with a menopausal patient with psychological symptoms, consider the following questions. Are the mood symptoms secondary to somatic hypoestrogenic symptoms? Is quality of life impaired by vasomotor symptoms, insomnia or urogenital atrophy? HRT, patient education and reassurance will be helpful.

Are the psychological symptoms a new occurrence or is there a previous history of psychiatric problems? The best predictor of the future course for most psychiatric illnesses is the past history. In the presence of a previous history, the treatment will depend on the nature of the specific problem and on the possible role played by any precipitating event. The treatment then should be specific for the underlying psychiatric problem, and a psychiatric referral or consultation should be considered.

If the emotional difficulties are new and persist after HRT has alleviated the hypoestrogenic symptoms, one would approach the patient as one would any patient presenting with an emotional problem – consider a psychiatric referral. Mental health professionals are best trained to evaluate and to treat individuals with emotional problems. This would be far superior to assuming that the patient has some kind of a 'chemical imbalance' and prescribing an antidepressant.

REFERENCES

1 Kaufert P, Gilbert P, Tate R: Defining menopausal status: The impact of longitudinal data. *Maturitas* 9: 217–226,1987.
2 Anderson E, Hamburger S, Liu JG, Rebar RW: Characteristics of menopausal women seeking assistance. *Am J Obstet Gynecol* 156: 428–433,1987.
3 Hagstad A, Janson P: The epidemiology of climacteric symptoms. *Acta Obs Gyn Scand* (suppl),134: 59–65,1986.
4 Warnock J: On some of the relationship between menstruation and insanity. *North Am Practitioner* 2: 49–59,1890.
5 Wilbrush J: La Menopausie – the birth of a syndrome. *Maturitas* 1: 145–151,1979.
6 Conklin WJ: Some neuroses of the menopause. *Trans Am Assoc Obstet Gynecol* 2: 301–311,1889.
7 Leake J: *Chronic or Slow Diseases Peculiar to Women*. London: Baldwin, 1777.
8 Meigs CD: *Women: Her Diseases and Remedies*. Philadelphia: Lea and Blanchard, 1851, pp. 38–45.
9 Shakespeare W: *Hamlet*. 1623. ed. Hoy C. New York: Norton, 1963.
10 Hoch A, MacCurdy JT: The prognosis of involutional melancholia. *Arch Neurol Psychiatry* 7: 1–17,1922.
11 Novak E: *Menstruation and Its Disorders*. New York: Appleton, 1923, pp. 146–149.
12 Redlich FC, Freedman DX: *The Theory and Practice of Psychiatry*. New York: Basic Books, 1966.
13 Roth M: The phenomenology of depressive states. *Can Psychiatr Assoc J* 4: 32–54,1959.
14 Gitlin MJ, Pasnau RO: Psychiatric syndromes linked to reproductive function in women: a review of current knowledge. *Am J Psychiatry* 146: 1413–1422,1989.
15 Matthews KA, Wing RR, Kullen LH, et al.: Influences of natural menopause on psychological characteristics and symptoms of middle-aged healthy women. *J Consult Clin Psychol* 58: 345–351,1990.
16 Weissman MM: The myth of involutional melancholia. *JAMA* 242: 742–744,1979.
17 Winokur G: Depression in menopause. *Am J Psychiatry* 130: 92–93,1973.
18 Hallstrom T, Samuelsson S: Mental health in the climacteric: the longitudinal study of women in Gothenburg. *Acta Obstet Gynecol Scand* 130: 13–18,1985.
19 Ballinger CB: Psychiatric aspects of the menopause. *Br J Psychiatry* 156: 773–787,1990.
20 McKinlay SM, Brambilla DJ, Pasner JG: *Maturitas* 14: 103–115,1992.
21 Myers JK, Weissman MM, Tischler GL, et al.: Six-month prevalence of psychiatric disorders in three communities. *Arch Gen Psychiatry* 41: 959–967,1984.
22 McKinlay SM, Jeffreys M: The menopausal syndrome. *Br J Preventive Social Med* 28: 108–115,1974.

23 Regier DA, Boyd JH, Burke JD, *et al.*: One month prevalence of mental disorders in the U.S. based on five Epidemiologic Catchment Area Sites. *Arch Gen Psychiatry* 45: 977–986,1988.

24 Kessler RC, McGonagle DA, Zhao S, *et al.*: Lifetime and 12-month prevalence of DSM-III-R psychiatric disorders in the U.S. *Arch Gen Psychiatry* 51: 8–19,1994.

25 Matthews KA: Myths and realities of the menopause. *Psychosom Med* 54: 1–9,1992.

26 Greene JG, Cooke DJ: Life stress and symptoms at the climacterium. *Br J Psychiatry* 136: 486–491,1980.

27 Jaszmann L, Van Lith ND, Zatt JCA: The perimenopausal symptoms. *Med Gynecology and Sociology* 4: 268–277,1969.

28 Barrett L, Cullis W, Fairfield L, *et al.*: Investigations of the menopause in 1000 women. *Lancet* 1: 106,1933.

29 Schmidt PJ, Rubinow DR: Menopause-related affective disorders: A justification for further study. *Am J Psych* 148: 844–852,1991.

30 American Psychiatric Association: *Diagnostic and Statistical Manual of Mental Disorders*. Fourth edition. Washington, DC: American Psychiatric Association, 1994.

31 Dennerstein L, Burrows GD, Hyman GJ, *et al.*: Hormone therapy and affect. *Maturitas* 1: 247–259,1979.

32 McEwen BS: The brain as a target organ of endocrine hormones. In Krieger DT, Hughes JS, eds. *Neuroendocrinology*. Sunderland, MA: Sinauer Assoc; 1980; pp. 33–42.

33 Luine VN, McEwen BS: Effect of estradiol on turnover of type A monoamine oxidase in brain. *J Neurochem* 28: 1221–1227,1977.

34 Aylward M: Plasma tryptophan levels and mental depression in postmenopausal subjects: effects of oral piperazine–oestrone sulphate. *IRCS Med Sci* 1: 30–34,1973.

35 Schildkraut JJ: The catecholamine hypothesis of affective disorders: a review of supporting evidence. *Am J Psychiatry* 122: 509–522,1965.

36 Luine VN, Khylchevaskaya RI, McEwen BS: Effect of gonadal steroids on activities of monoamine oxidase and cholin acetylase in rat brain. *Brain Res* 86: 293–306,1975.

37 Bartus RT, Dean RL, Beer B, Lippa AS: The cholinergic hypothesis of memory function. *Science* 217: 408–417,1982.

38 Beer AE, Billingham RE: Maternal immunological mechanisms during pregnancy. *Ciba Found Symp* 64: 293–322,1979.

39 Magos AL, Brewster E, Singh R, O'Dowd T, Bincat M, Studd JWW: The effects of norethisterone in postmenopausal women on oestrogen replacement therapy: A model for the premenstrual syndrome. *Br J Obstet Gynecol* 93: 1290,1986.

40 Holst J, Backstrom T, Hammerback S, von Schoultz B: Progesterone addition during oestrogen replacement therapy – effects on vasomotor symptoms and mood. *Maturitas* 11: 13,1989.

41 Sherwin BB: Estrogen and/or androgen replacement therapy and cognitive functioning in surgically menopausal women. *Psychoendocrinology* 13: 345–357,1988.

42 Kleiber E, Broverman: Estrogen therapy for severe persistent depressions in women. *Arch Gen Psychiatry* 36: 550,1974.

43 Schneider MA, Brotherton PL, Hailes J: The effect of exogenous oestrogens on depression in menopausal women. *Med J Aust* 2: 162–163,1977.

44 Oppenheim G, Zohar J, Shapiro B, *et al.*: The rates of estrogen in treating resistant depression. In Zohar J, Belmaker RH, eds. *Treating Resistant Depression*. Boston: PMA Publishing, 1987, pp. 357–363.

45 Sherwin BB, Gelfand MM: Sex steroids and affect in the surgical menopause: A double-blind crossover study. *Psychoendocrinology* 10: 325–335,1985.

46 Sherwin BB: Affective changes with estrogen and androgen replacement therapy in surgically menopausal women. *J Aff Dis* 14: 177–187,1988.

47 Sherwin BB: The impact of different doses of estrogen and progestin on mood and sexual behavior in postmenopausal women. *J Clin Endocrinol Metab* 72: 336–343,1991.

48 Schiff I, Regestein Q, Tulchinsky D, *et al.*: Effects of estrogens on sleep and psychological state of hypogonadal women. *JAMA* 242: 2405–2407,1979.

49 Campbell S, Whitehead M: Oestrogen therapy and the menopausal syndrome. *Clin Obstet Gynecol* 4: 31–47,1977.

50 Erlik Y, Tataryn IV, Meldrum DR, Lomax P, Bajorek JG, Judd HL: Association of waking episodes with menopausal hot flushes. *JAMA* 245: 1741–1744,1981.

51 Skegg DC, Doll R, Perry J: Use of medicines in general practice. *BMJ* 1: 1561–1563,1977.

52 Molnar GW: Body temperatures during menopausal hot flashes. *J Appl Physiol* 38: 499–503,1975.

53 McKinlay J, McKinlay S, Brambilla D: The relative contributions of endocrine changes and social circumstances to depression in mid-aged women. *J Health Soc Beh* 28: 345–363,1987.

54 McKinlay J, McKinlay S, Brambilla D: Health status and utilization behavior associated with menopause. *Am J Epidemiol* 125: 110–121,1987.

55 Greene JG: Psychosocial influences and life events at the time of the menopause. In: Formanek R, ed. *The Meaning of Menopause: Historical, Medical and Clinical Perspectives*. Hillsdale, New Jersey: The Analytic Press, 1990: 79–115.

56 Erikson EH: Eight ages of man. In: *Childhood and Society*. New York: W.W. Norton, 1963, pp. 268–269.

57 Newgarten B: *Middle Age and Aging*. Chicago, IL: University of Chicago Press, 1978.

58 Colarusso C, Nemiroff R, Zucherman S: Female mid-life issues in prose and poetry. In: Colarusso C, Nemiroff R, eds. *Adult Development*. New York: Plenum Press, 1981, pp. 141–165.

59 Notman M: Mid-life concerns of women: Implications of the menopause. *Am J Psych* 136: 1270,1979.

60 Barnett R, Baruch G: Women in the middle years: Conceptions and misconceptions. In: Willams J, ed. *Psychology of Women: Selected Readings*. New York: Norton, 1978, pp. 479–487.

61 Notman M: Mid-life concerns of women: Implications of the menopause. In: Nadelson C, Notman M, eds. *The Woman Patient: Concepts of Femininity and the Life Cycle*. Vol. 2. New York: Plenum Press, 1978, pp. 135–144.

62 Eisenberg L: Medicine – molecular, monetary, or more than both. *JAMA* 274: 331–334,1995.

63 Engel GL: The need for a new medical model: A challenge for biomedicine. *Science* 196: 129,1977.

64 Winokur G, Cadoret R: The irrelevance of the menopause to depressive illness. In: Sachar EJ, ed. *Topics in Psychoendocrinology*. New York: Grune & Stratton, 1975.

65 Tallmer Margot: Empty nest syndrome: Possibility or despair. In: Bernay T, Cantor, D, eds. *The Psychology of Today's Woman: New Psychoanalytic Perspectives*.Hillsdale, NJ: The Analytic Press, 1986, pp. 231–252.

66 Campagnoli *et al.*: Climacteric symptoms according to body weight in women of different socio-economic groups. *Maturitas* 3: 279–287,1981.

67 Hunter M, Battersby R, Whitehead M: Relationships between psychological symptoms, somatic complaints and menopausal status. *Maturitas* 8: 217–228,1986.

68 Polit D, Larocco S: Social and psychological correlates of the menopausal symptoms. *Psychosom Med* 42: 335–345,1980.

69 Abe T, Mortisuka T: A case control study on climacteric symptoms and complaints of Japanese women by symptomatic type for psychological variables. *Maturitas* 8: 255–265,1986.

70 Datan N: Aging into transitions: Cross-cultural perspectives on women at midlife. In: Formanek R, ed. *The Meaning of Menopause: Historical, Medical and Clinical Perspectives*. Hillsdale, NJ: The Analytic Press, 1990.

71 Flint M: Cross-cultural factors that affect age of menopause. *Consensus on Menopause Research of*

the Proceedings of the 1st International Congress on Menopause. Baltimore: University Park Press, 1976, p. 73.

72 Beyene Y: Cultural significance and physiological manifestations of menopause. A biocultural analysis. *Cult Med Psychiat* 10: 47–71,1986.

73 Lock M: Ambiguities of aging. *Cult Med Psychiat* 10: 23–46,1986.

74 Davidson JM: The psychobiology of sexual experience. *Maturitas* 7: 193–201,1985.

75 Pfeiffer E, Verwoerdt A, Davis GC: Sexual behavior in middle life. *Am J Psychiatry* 129: 82–88,1972.

76 Newman G, Nichols CR: Sexual activities and attitudes in older persons. *JAMA* 173(1): 117,1960.

77 Bachmann GA, Leiblum S: Sexual expression in menopausal women. *Med Asp Hum Sex* 15: 96b–96h,1981.

78 Leiblum S, Swartzman L: Women's attitudes toward the menopause: An update. *Maturitas* 8: 47–56,1986.

79 Brecher EM: *Love, Sex and Aging*. Boston: Little Brown, 1984, pp. 311–345.

80 Willson JR: The aging woman. In Sciarra JJ, ed. *Gynecology and Obstetrics*. Philadelphia: Harper and Row, 1987, pp. 1–12.

81 Sherwin BB, Gelfand MM: Androgen enhances sexual motivation in females. *Psychosom Med* 47: 351–379,1985.

82 Rako S: Testosterone deficiency and supplementation for women: Matters of sexuality and health. *Psychiatric Annals* 29: 23–26, 1999.

83 Berlin FS, Meinecke CF: Treatment of sex offenders with antiandrogenic medication. *Am J Psychiatry* 138: 601–607,1981.

84 Dennerstein L, Burrows GD, Wood C, Hyman G: Hormones and sexuality: effect of estrogen and progesterone. *Obstet Gynecol* 56: 316–322,1980.

85 Sherwin BB: The impact of different doses of estrogen and progestin on mood and sexual behavior in postmenopausal women. *J Clin Endocrinol Metab* 72: (2)336–343,1991.

86 Smith RNJ, Studd JWW: Estrogens and depression in women. In: Lobo RA, ed. *Treatment of the Postmenopausal Woman: Basic and Clinical Aspects*. New York: Raven Press, 1994, pp. 129–135.

87 Arpels JC: The female brain hypoestrogenic continuum from the premenstrual syndrome to menopause. A hypothesis and review of supporting data. *J Reprod Med* 41: 633–639,1996.

4

Sexuality

RICHARD J HAM

INTRODUCTION

Many clinicians, even in this enlightened age, are uncomfortable dealing with issues of sexuality in their patients, both young and old, but especially the latter. Yet it is clear that any physician (not just gynecologists and other primary care physicians) will be involved in diagnostic and treatment decisions that are liable to affect their patients' sexual function and capacity.[1]

Part of the tremendous social and medical impact of AIDS/HIV has been a profound effect on sexual mores; a changed attitude, perhaps a new conservatism, towards sexual continence and abstinence and the dangers of promiscuity.[2,3] There has also developed a generally better understanding of homosexual relationships, both male and female, and of the potential stability of such relationships.

Despite this enforced increased awareness of the centrality of sexual function to medical problems, still only a minority of existing clinicians are trained and comfortable with discussing heterosexual functionality and the way it changes in different illness states, at different levels of health status and at different ages and phases in our patients' lives. Clinicians need to be able to identify the primary sexual disorders, such as erectile dysfunction, vaginismus, premature ejaculation and anorgasmia. Having identified these, clinicians need active contact and professional rapport with individuals skilled and trained in the sexual therapy that is generally indicated in such disorders. And they will have to be comfortable about their role, which at a minimum includes an evaluation for medical factors contributing to such problems.

As individuals age and ongoing health problems occur, the clinician can be astoundingly helpful in preserving sexual function by considering it in the many illnesses and therapies that will influence it and by discussing, when necessary, appropriate positions for sexual activity. Sexual positioning may well be compromised in many of the illnesses that afflict us with increasing frequency as we grow older, such as osteoarthritis, cardiac problems and lung disease.

This chapter will summarize what is known about common changes in sexual function with increasing age, after the menopause and on into old age. It will also describe the principles of identifying the primary sexual disorders, with suggestions as to the physician's appropriate approach to the medical management and therapy, where indicated, of such issues. It will identify a number of medical areas, including those separate from the specialized attention of gynecologists, where sexuality should be introduced as an issue and specific advice given. It is important for gynecologists to be familiar with these latter illnesses, since increasingly gynecologists are primary care physicians. They will therefore need to have a primary care overview of non-gynecologic illnesses and their implications for patients.

UNIQUENESS OF THE SEXUAL RESPONSE

There is perhaps no area of human activity more profoundly influenced by many different factors than sexuality. The unpredictable nature of any individual's sexual development, the way in which an individual's sexuality develops through experiences over time, interacting with circumstances, culture, education and physique, interacting with changing societal mores, with the differing expectation of peers and partners, and the clearly unique level of importance that sexuality assumes in any individual's life are but a selection of the range of influences whose aggregate effect, when analyzed, can helpfully explain the sexuality and the sexual problems, if any, of each individual.

This huge range of influences demonstrate the dangers of generalization, of assumptions, of 'norms': each person is sexually unique.

In an attempt to give some shape to this huge subject in the context of a brief review that will be useful for clinicians, I have divided these influences into categories, subheadings under which the clinical implications are summarized.

ATTITUDES AND PREJUDICE

The view that sex after reproductive capacity, and especially on into old age, is ridiculous and pathetic has been extant since ancient times.[4] Humankind is unique in maintaining sexual function for a long period of life after the natural capacity for reproduction. But then, humankind is somewhat unique in having an extended period of nonreproductive life, against a background, generally, of coupling partnerships (or at least an ambition to be a partner in a couple!), generally with that relationship being more/or less the exclusive sexual one for both partners.

However, as Masters and Johnson, wrote decades ago, 'human sexual needs are life-long'. Their studies of sexuality in volunteer older couples confirmed that continuing sexuality, both heterosexual and homosexual is possible, commonplace, and important and significant to many individuals as they age.[5–7] Age alone is certainly not a barrier to sexual fulfilment in men and in women. To clinicians, the important point is that with increasing age, medical problems start to become barriers to sexual response, so clinicians in particular have a special responsibility to assist those who wish to maintain a sexual life to do so.

One of the consequences of the attitudes that sexuality in old age is somehow unnatural is that many physicians and other clinicians are uncomfortable introducing the subject of sexuality, in part because of their own embarrassment, but in part because they fear embarrassing an older person or offending sensibilities; because much sexual unhappiness is unreported, it is therefore unaddressed.

These attitudinal difficulties are reinforced by the physical changes that occur in many as they age and which specifically affect sexual response: whereas fit older individuals have sexual responses very much like those of younger people, certain changes are common, and the fact is that the overall 'average' male changes in sexual response can easily be interpreted as demonstrating failing sexual prowess or pending impotence, whereas changes in women mostly tend to produce discomfort, dyspareunia, as well as diminished actual sexual sensation. But what is known about the changing sexual response in men and women will be described later. The point is that there are changes which occur in many men and women, both around the time of the menopause and then increasingly into old age, that can easily add to the attitudinal conflicts and lead to a downward spiral of diminishing sexual activity for avoidable reasons.

The reader must not assume here that there is any sense of advocacy to indicate that sexuality *ought* to be part of all relationships with increasing age. We have evidence since ancient times of the potentially positive psychological effects of abstinence, and sometimes the most successful adaptation is to give up on an activity which is causing difficulty, discomfort or embarrassment, or emotional upset to patients or their partners. Such adaptation underlies one of the recognized and described patterns of adaptation to old age in general, and may be normal and satisfactory. What sometimes goes wrong is that one partner is comfortable with the giving up, and the other is not. This may or may not be a factor in the considerably more troublesome sexual acting out that widowed older men tend to produce in terms of disruptive sexual behaviours in nursing homes.[8,9]

And what is the clinician's role in this subject of importance for every patient? Perhaps most vital is that the clinician must express an appropriately positive view about sexuality, recognizing its significance, asking about it, making it possible for patients to freely discuss it, and conveying a realistic approach to it. The fact that many older individuals experience lifelong satisfactory sexuality, the fact that sexual function often improves dramatically in the perimenopausal period as individuals become more confident of their own sexuality and response, and the fact that professional help is available if difficulties arise and really can work, provided it is offered in a timely, positive manner and problems are not allowed to become irremediable through chronicity – all these facts need to be appreciated by the clinician and conveyed to the patient. In an area of human performance where failure and negativity so easily translates into physical difficulties and self-fulfilling prophecy, assuming that sexuality is bound to be problematic in the time of the menopause and bound to be increasingly unsatisfactory and unpleasant with increasing age is just plain wrong. Yet many of us, clinicians and nonclinicians, do not know this; we may convey negativity and confirm negativity by the way we ask questions or fail to, or by the way we too rapidly reassure or dismiss our patients' concerns when they are expressed.

Thus how to overcome some of these problems clinically includes encouraging far more openness in preappointment questionnaires, for example, about sexuality, as well as discussions about it during the course of history and physical examination. But clinicians have to get comfortable enough with this and sensitive enough to patients responses that they also 'hear' when the individual does not wish to discuss sexuality.

PRIMARY SEXUAL DISORDERS

Although this is not the place to give a detailed description of the sexual disorders, it must be emphasized that, at any age, certain primary sexual disorders can occur, and it is unfortunately true that many clinicians are unprepared to recognize and discuss even these.[10] So they will be briefly described here.

Premature ejaculation

Whereas changes in old age in men mostly tend to counteract this common phenomenon, it most certainly can occur. It may be a special problem in new relationships, or in ones associated with excess emotionality. Clinicians and sexual therapists can teach techniques to distract, delay and influence physically (penile squeeze) to reduce this happening.

Primary erectile dysfunction

Clinicians recognize that this can be a symptom of diabetic neuropathy, but demonstrations of improved sexual performance in individuals felt definitely to have diabetic neuropathy as the reason for failed erection demonstrates the interaction of psychological and partner factors in the production of this.[11] Sexual therapy should always be offered, even if investigations suggest that there may truly be neurologic deterioration, such as, for example, a history of open prostatectomy or other bladder surgery, and/or the presence of diabetes and other signs of diabetic neuropathy.

Vaginismus

Psychological and painful stimuli, especially including local pain in the genital tract, predispose to this common phenomenon and, combined with dryness and atrophy (see below), one can see how this can become a common syndrome in the perimenopausal and postmenopausal period. Multiple factors may be involved, and the clinician's help in controlling local and medical factors, and advising or seeking formal sexual therapy if necessary to assist in the gentling of technique that is necessary to overcome it, can be curative.

Anorgasmia

Orgasmic dysfunction occurs in both men and women. Its interrelationship with estrogen and progesterone levels remains elusively unclear, since actual performance change as a result of hormonal change is unpredictable. Whereas it is recognized that progesterone deficiency can produce orgasmic pain, it is possible that hormonal influences might be helpful in enhancing or reacquiring orgasmic response. However, such research is difficult and indeed controversial, and it is not clear that the risks outweigh the benefits of using hormonal supplementation in these ways. What is recognized is that orgasmic dysfunction will frequently respond to traditional sexual therapeutic techniques, especially if both partners can be involved.

In men, there may be anorgasmia, or there may be failed ejaculatory function despite orgasm. Masters and Johnson state emphatically that the recognition of anejaculatory orgasm as an acceptable and normal phenomenon with increasing age in men can be the key to continuing satisfactory sexual relationships in many couples.[5]

THE STAGES OF HUMAN SEXUAL RESPONSE

Human sexual response is generally divided into four stages, and the recognition that these are separate stages forms the basis for most therapeutic approaches. Dysfunction in one area need not necessarily produce dysfunction in all the others, although this often will happen. Most therapists will start their history by dividing up the response of the individual and/or of the couple's sexual activity into these stages in order to define where the problem is. Therapy will then focus on maintaining the successful stages and working on the unsuccessful stages.

The four phases are:

- excitation
- plateau
- orgasm
- resolution

Heterosexual and homosexual relationships both involve the same phases, as does masturbatory activity. The importance of masturbation as a sexual comfort to lonely individuals, the separated and widowed must be recognized. Failing to allow privacy for individual sexual activity in the institutionalized is inhumane.[12,13] This author had the early experience of proposing catheterization for an elderly man, bed-bound, hemiplegic in his remaining side with a one-sided amputation: a very difficult nursing situation, and a tough existence. Fortunately, he had the courage to tell me that a catheter would interfere with one of his remaining pleasures, one that I had not considered (masturbation), even though I would have characterized my concern for him as to give him as much quality of life and experience as possible despite his disabilities.

OPPORTUNITIES FOR SEXUAL ACTIVITY

The pressures of parenting, careers, travel and absences, and the necessity for abstinence during illness and other separations clarify the need to adapt one's sexual mores and expectations to the circumstances of life. The couple who can be candid with one another about their sexual needs will approach the challenging time of perimenopause and the even more challenging time of old age together much better prepared than individuals lacking such openness of communication.

As subsequent sections discuss, many and varied changes take place both physically and in terms of physiological variations in sexual response as a result of the change in hormonal influences (and the change in psychological and often circumstantial influences) of the perimenopause. In some women, menstrual and other hormonally influenced physical changes may well create a distaste for sexual matters for a time. In others, sexual appetite and drive may increase. Recognition that such changes in sexual performance and expectation do occur during the perimenopause is vital. In any relationship, both partners need to adapt! If the couple have handled periods of abstinence or periods of greatly increased activity, they may be well prepared.

It is important to realize that the perimenopause often coincides with a period of intense, ambitious work, by both partners in the relationship. Many careers are at their peak at the period of the perimenopause. Thus both partners will be potentially in situations where flexibility for all of life's arrangements, including those for sex, cannot be achieved.

Further after the menopause, widowhood, much more common in women than men of course, deprives women of social and sexual contact. Society is still arranged so that it is often more difficult for the widowed woman to reestablish social contacts.

In addition, Masters and Johnson describe the 'widows and widowers syndromes' to characterize the difficulties of restarting a sexual relationship in a late-life remarriage.[5] There are many opportunities for the sensitive clinician to be medically useful in such situations. Whereas men may readapt easily to sexual activity, in the postmenopausal woman, altered vaginal tone, viscosity of secretions and actual vaginal narrowing may be physical factors to consider, and even plastic surgical interventions or progressive dilation may be needed.

Later in life, the rekindling of romantic social and sexual interest between the long-widowed will often produce problems in the younger remaining family, not just because of prejudice or feelings about sex, but because of genuine fears about the loss of the estate and other testamentary considerations.

PSYCHOLOGICAL ISSUES

Later sections will summarize the physical changes that often take place. Women tend to experience more discomfort with attempted intercourse, while men experience changes that can be misinterpreted as pending impotence, and these changes feed into negative thoughts about sexuality and sexual image with increasing age.

It has been argued that many women give up the sexual role with relief, that a fear of rejection and changed self-image leads to an adaptive activity; withdrawing from sex.[14] It is certainly true that society regards aging men as more sexually attractive than aging women. Nonetheless, aging women have their own needs of sexual fulfilment, as is evident from many sources.

Sexuality relates to self-image, to an individual's sense of achievement and involvement. Thus sexual difficulties may start when the professional, ego-enhancing roles of working life are given up, as occurs at retirement.

An additional factor of retirement is that expectations for the relationship, including sexual aspects of it, may increase. Difficulties will be highlighted by the extra time available, and that anticipated pleasant retirement may then be a disappointment ('I married him for better or for worse but not for lunch' – Anonymous).[1]

With increasing age and increasing physical problems comes the fear of harm being caused by intercourse. This is particularly identified following cardiovascular events, such as myocardial infarction and cerebrovascular accident. It is here that the clinician's role in reassuring the individual and counseling about the appropriate resumption of sexual activity after such major illness is important. It has been shown that specifically adding sexual counseling after a myocardial infarction improves well-being in a number of parameters.[15]

But there are psychological factors which are positive also. Once the menopause is firmly established, the fear of pregnancy is removed. Possibly for the first time in life it will not be necessary to use physical barriers, and sexual enjoyment and sensation can then be enhanced.

Around this time (the perimenopause), many individuals are experiencing the absence of children or other young people in the home, increasing the opportunity for sexual activity. There may be increasing independence to schedule one's own time, and the opportunity then to schedule sexual activity along with other enjoyable activities at optimal times, rather than merely when they can be fitted in.

CHANGES IN FEMALE SEXUAL FUNCTION AND RESPONSE

Most of the changes that have been defined as occurring 'normally' with increasing age, and which start within a few years of the menopause and increase with increasing age, are in fact related to estrogen loss (Table 4.1). Many of them could be prevented, or at least reduced or postponed, by estrogen therapy. There are many reasons to consider estrogen therapy in the postmenopausal phase, and other sections in this book address the many advantages.[16,17] One is a reduction in the changes induced by lack of estrogen, which causes many of the 'normal' changes of the physical status of the female genital tract with increasing age that are described by Masters and Johnson.[6]

These changes include reduced vascularity and fat in the walls of the vulva, with a vulva and vagina that is smaller, smoother and thinner. There is often laxity of the vaginal walls, which reduces sexual sensation for both partners. Yet the vagina itself, unstimulated is frequently narrower. It is known that the physiological responses during the four phases (excitement, plateau, orgasm and resolution) are changed, within generally less variation in vaginal size during intercourse. Overall, there appears to be reduction in the length and intensity of each of the four phases. As mentioned before, progesterone deficiency is thought to be the initiator of the orgasmic pain experienced by some women. Painful orgasms should lead to consideration of progesterone supplementation.

The classic change of atrophic vaginitis, although common, should not be considered a normal phenomenon. It is caused by lack of estrogen. Clearly, the vaginal wall in atrophic vaginitis, with its bleeding, rawness and fragility, and its contribution to dyspareunia, is a disincentive to satisfactory sexual relationships.

In addition, there is a drying up of vaginal secretions postmenopausally and as one ages. That is why lubrication alone (as in earlier ages) is a frequently important, simple, sexual aid. Therapeutically, it must be remembered that non-water-soluble lubricants such as

Table 4.1 *Genital changes in the average elderly female*

Reduced vascularity and fat content of the vaginal walls
Reduced size of vulva and vagina
Stickier, reduced secretions
Thinner, more lax vaginal walls
Less variability of vaginal size during intercourse
Shorter, less intense orgasms
Reduced sexual response in all four phases
Painful orgasms in some
Atrophic vaginitis, with bleeding, infection, and dyspareunia in some

petroleum jelly are altogether less satisfactory than water-soluble (and therefore washable) lubricants such as K-Y jelly and other proprietary lubricants (which can also be warmed before use – very helpful as a sexual aid!). But any lubricant has tremendous utility in maintaining sexual activity in the perimenopausal phase and on into old age.

The implications of these changes for the relevant physical examination in any individual experiencing sexual difficulties are obvious. The finding of dryness should lead to discussion about lubrication and how to increase it, including perhaps the issues of sexual technique to increase secretions, or oral sex to improve lubrication. But these maybe enormous changes in technique that cannot be achieved in a conservative older individual. The perimenopausal person, however, may still be 'young' enough to adapt!

CHANGES IN THE MALE GENITAL TRACT WITH INCREASING AGE

The likely contemporary partner of the perimenopausal female – and most men at around that age – has sexual responses very similar to those occurring in younger age groups. The degree of adaptation that the male partner will be able to achieve will be important, however, and as age increases, the fact that many phenomena have been described as being very common in aged males should be known. Misinterpretation of the common changes of aging that occur in male sexual response undoubtedly leads to many assumptions of pending impotence, which easily become self-fulfilling.

Masters and Johnson describe what they call 'first-time failure': one failed sexual encounter leads to a downward spiral, with each attempt fraught with self-doubt and therefore with unsatisfactory results.[5] This 'first-time failure' phenomenon often occurs after some transient issue (for example, overindulgence in alcohol or caffeine, both of which can inhibit sexual response), which is especially regrettable. Sexual activity cannot be 'forced': performance anxiety reduces the chances of it coming out right.

Published observations of the sexual responses of aging men are perhaps misleading.[6,7] It is almost certain that these changes should not appropriately be described as 'normal', since physically fit, or physically more-fit-than-average individuals such as elderly athletic men, appear to have normal sexual responses. However, the changes summarized in Table 4.2 are relevant, for they are the sexual changes that many men experience with increasing age, but generally not until their sixties and seventies or even beyond. The main point is that the changes overall can be misinterpreted as impotence.

All phases of the sexual response can be affected, with the excitation phase and the achievement of erection being generally slower and weaker; and in many older men, maximal erection occurs only just before ejaculation. The importance of this in relation to reducing sexual sensation in both partners is obvious. It is also frequently found that the sensation of ejaculatory inevitability is reduced, that is, there is less forewarning or less

Table 4.2 *Genital changes in the average elderly male*

Reduced penile sensitivity
Slower, weaker erection
Reduced ejaculatory volume
Anejaculatory orgasm
Reduced forewarning of ejaculation
Speedier detumescence
Increased refractory period

awareness of ejaculation being about to take place. This is the opposite of descriptions in the *Kama Sutra* and other ancient texts on sexuality of improved sexual function in the older man because of improved control (in part secondary to reduced sensation). Clearly, the individual with less awareness of his own sexual response and sensations will be less able to organize sexual activity so as to give pleasure to both himself and his partner. Ejaculatory volume is generally reduced, and the phenomenon of orgasm sometimes occurring without ejaculation at all (often with the contractions associated, but not with the actual ejaculation of semen) is obviously important. While it makes no difference to the completion of the sexual act and its potential psychological satisfaction, many men will be worried about the absence of ejaculation, and again, a self-fulfilling prophecy of reduced potency may be the result. Both partners need to know about this.

The phase of resolution, with detumescence of the penis, is usually quicker than in younger men, and a further sexual change affects the responsiveness after the completion of sexual activity: the so-called 'refractory period', which is the time that elapses before ejaculation can be achieved again (not just erection), is often prolonged in older men; it can be up to 12 or 24 hours.

There is evidence of reduction of sensory input in many situations with increasing age, and the implication is that penile sensitivity is also reduced. This can combine with vaginal laxity in the partner to reduce sexual sensation for both. Changes in technique, with increased manual stimulation by either partner, may well be necessary.

In summary, frequently found male changes include experiencing a brief orgasm with little sensation and no ejaculation, with a quick loss of erection, all of this causing less sexual sensation, and in circumstances that feel like reduced control, with ejaculation being able to be reachieved after a longer interval than in earlier life.

PHYSICAL ILLNESS AND SEXUAL RESPONSE

The gynecologist is, by definition, closely involved in assessing physical changes that can affect sexuality. However, if gynecologists take on broader primary care roles, they will need to 'cast their net wider' in terms of considering, as all primary care physicians should, the sexual implications of many of the illnesses we manage.

Gynecological abnormalities are bound to have sexual significance. Anything that causes discomfort, limits sexual activity, reduces sensation, or in any way changes the response of the physical relationships, whether a change in the male or female, has significant sexual implications that should be discussed by the clinician.

Urinary incontinence, a common phenomenon and one that is frequently not fully described and discussed with the physician, has sexual implications as well. Perineal hygiene, bladder emptying, sexual position and so forth are all important. The full urinary bladder may modify or increase sexual sensation.

In the male, prostatectomy may well affect ejaculatory volume, or there may be reverse ejaculation causing a form of anejaculatory orgasm. Even the periurethral approach (TURP) to prostatectomy can cause nerve damage and affect function. Surgery or illness associated with any of the interconnecting male or female sexual organs always includes sexual implications, which should be discussed. Even medical problems that are close by, such as hernia repair, should properly involve counselling about sexuality.

The sexual implication of mastectomy are well recognized, although the tendency now to use less mutilating surgery, and also sometimes to do breast reconstruction when more than a lumpectomy is needed, will help.

The sexual implications of colostomy are well recognized, and colostomy nurses are frank about discussing it. Modern colostomy and barrier techniques can ensure that there is no odor, which would obviously be a disincentive to sexual activity. Unfortunately, we do not have the same discussion so consistently in relation to the many other surgeries which also have sexual implications. Any individual undergoing abdominal surgery needs to know when sexual activity can be recommenced, otherwise they will fear to do so.

Osteoarthritis, the commonest chronic condition in the world, will characteristically cause reduced ability to rotate the hips and bend the knees when those joints are affected, as they commonly are. In either partner, this will affect sexual positioning, sexual expression and sexual function. Osteoarthritis is but one reason why clinicians must be adept at discussing sexual positioning in relation to a person's specific disabilities.

Just as gynecologists and all primary care physicians must become more used to doing their gynecologic examinations in the left lateral position in order to make it comfortable and possible for an individual with advanced arthritis of the hips or knees to actually undergo that examination, so similarly positioning needs to be adapted for sexual activity (see below).

Many other symptoms can influence sexual function. An individual with chronic lung disease for example, may find it uncomfortable to be recumbent for sexual activity, and may need a different position.

Diabetic patients recognize that diabetic neuropathy can cause sexual changes, especially in men. The fact that counseling can overcome the physical effects of even established confirmed neuropathy has been emphasized above.

MEDICATIONS AND SEX

'First do no harm' is part of the Hippocratic oath, and it is generally interpreted nowadays as meaning that medications can harm patients – and it is certainly true that they can.[18]

So, too, can other 'medications' available over the counter and through the liquor store be harmful: alcohol, the most easily available psychotropic in the world, will generally diminish sexual performance and reduce skills as well. It has a role in 'first-time failure' described above. Caffeine, another easily available stimulant, and even the stimulant decongestant, pseudoephedrine, can cause diminished sexual performance.

Many medications are available over the counter that modify the sexual response. All of the antihistamines and many decongestant cough mixtures which contain antihistamines actually have powerful sedative and anticholinergic effects that can directly affect sexual function in a negative way.

The H_2 blockers, including cimetidine and many others, are now available over the counter. It is well-recognized that they can diminish sexual performance and response.

Virtually all antihypertensive drugs, with the possible exception of the calcium channel blockers and ACE inhibitors, can interfere with sexual functioning. Many antidepressants will interfere with sexual functioning, despite the fact that reduced libido is a symptom of depression which obviously may respond to antidepressant treatment.

Many analgesics, not just the narcotics, can reduce sexual response. Digoxin, a medication frequently continued unnecessarily in individuals who do not need it for its inotropic effects, can also reduce sexual response. Other medications that have been implicated include anticancer medications in general, the anticonvulsant phenytoin and the anti-parkinsonian medication levodopa (even in its combined form with carbidopa, Sinemet).

The ability of NSAIDs to diminish the sexual response and cause anorgasmia is well recognized. Naproxen was the first to be so implicated. These medications are frequently available over the counter, and are now widely recommended for headaches, premenstrual syndrome, gynecological cramps, and fever control, as well as their original indication for arthritic pain.

Many other medications not listed here can have sexual effects, and the rule remains that if there is a change in a person's sexual responsiveness, and if it coincides with a change in medication, the first assumption is that the medication may be the cause, and it should be discontinued if possible.

SEXUAL POSITIONING

To be an effective primary care physician to the older individual and the perimenopausal couple, sexual positions need to be able to be discussed.

Although physical limitations on sexual position are relatively rare in the perimenopausal phase, some individuals with chronic lung disease and arthritis will already be having problems by that stage, and may need advice. Certainly, sexual positioning is one important method whereby sexual activity may be able to be continued despite challenging problems such as congestive heart failure, chronic lung disease, osteoarthritis and other issues.[1,11]

For many individuals as they become more fragile or if they are unfit secondary to deconditioning or illness, a useful sexual position is to have both partners lying on their sides, torsos facing one another and legs intertwined, allowing them to be recumbent, and allowing easy access to one another sexually, without the necessity of supporting the weight on the forearms. More challenging is the individual who cannot lie flat, in which case sexual activity can be achieved in the sitting position, and whereas this may not seem very original to modern couples nowadays, to many older people it is quite a revolution to think in terms of intercourse with one partner sitting over the end of a bed, the other partner kneeling or perhaps sitting supported, so as to provide sexual access to one another.

Female superior, lateral positioning with both partners on their sides, or female facedown, male superior entering the partner from behind, may be useful for medical, not just sensual reasons.

Continuing sexual activity with increasing age, if there is disability, is undoubtedly dependent in part on an imaginative approach to sexual repositioning. Clinicians being able frankly to describe different sexual positions will greatly help the couple to overcome their difficulties.

INTERVENTIONS AND THERAPIES

Firstly, a preventive approach is best. The clinician who introduces sexual issues in situations where they are bound to be a problem (after myocardial infarction, after stroke, during the process of gynecological surgery, for example) will prevent a lot of problems!

The clinician must express his or her willingness to discuss sexual issues. Including such issues in preappointment questionnaires, as well as during routine history and physical examinations by both the clinician and his or her nurse practitioner and nurse, encourages the thought that sexuality is a natural part of health, a part in which the clinician has an interest and will be helpful.

However, no clinician, unless especially interested, is going to be able to devote the necessary time completely to treat some of the sexual problems that will be unearthed by such a proactive approach. So all primary care clinicians should establish professional rapport with one or more certified sexual therapists and/or other local experts, so that they have the referral network for any sexual problems that need more than the simple advice, reassurance and medical approaches that are implied in this chapter.

A certified sexual therapist will be confident in dealing with one or both partners, issues of homosexual and heterosexual sex, safe-sex issues and appropriate barriers, and the management of the primary sexual disorders, some of which are briefly summarized above. A sexual therapist could be very useful to help overcome the problems of the late-life remarriage or late-life first-time marriage.

Clinicians should realize that it has been convincingly demonstrated that even simply taking a sexual history can in itself be therapeutic, and in fact a very small amount of educational input can make a very profound difference.[19] Clinicians often hesitate to bring up issues where they feel they are opening up something that they cannot handle – which is why one's own referral network needs to be organized.

Other expertise that may be required includes the urologist and/or other male urologic tract surgeon for problems that may be found if the male partner is examined. Sometimes phimosis or balanitis is found in the noncircumcised male, for example, or other abnormalities in the male genitalia that somehow have been previously tolerated.

Some generalizations about therapeutic techniques should be made that apply to perimenopausal sexuality and to the problems that will arise more with increasing age:

1 Approach the sexual activity when fresh and refreshed, after a good night's sleep, and generally in the mornings (unless that is when arthritis is a problem, or one of the partners is a depressive and has diurnal variation).
2 Lubrication is essential. Estrogen replacement can sometimes achieve it, but sometimes other lubricants, preferably water-soluble heatable ones, can be astonishingly helpful and should be incorporated into one's individual sexual techniques.
3 There is often a clear need for increased stimulation of each other by both partners, and this may require changes in technique.
4 Full sexual intercourse should not always be the consequence of warmth or an embrace. Particularly if there is performance anxiety, or some insecurity in the relationship, it may be hardly possible for one to touch the other without feeling sexually challenged. Separating sex from the warmth and security of a hug needs to be achieved. The human need for sensual closeness and warmth is not entirely sexual!
5 If it is not being used for other reasons, estrogen replacement or estrogen vaginally can be astonishingly helpful for the sore dyspareunic rawness that many older women have to endure.
6 Unless both partners understand the average changes that take place, they will not be able to adapt completely to sexuality as they age.
7 Be prepared to counsel the situation where only one partner is concerned about sexuality, and the other is comfortable with the degree of 'giving up' that may have taken place.
8 It may be reasonable to discuss masturbation, erotic stimulation and other things that can be associated with guilt.

DEPRESSION AND SEXUALITY

Depression is an extremely common illness at all ages, often associated with the physical and emotional swings of the perimenopause, but also occurring with increasing prevalence

Table 4.3 *Criteria for major depression (DSM-IV)*

Depressed mood or loss of interest or pleasure in most or all usual activities plus at least four of these symptoms, all of this occurring for at least two weeks:
- Changes in appetite or weight
- Disturbed sleep
- Motor agitation or retardation
- Fatigue or loss of energy
- Feelings of worthlessness, self-reproach, or excessive guilt
- Suicidal thinking or attempts
- Difficulty with thinking or concentration

After DSM-IV, 1994

as age increases. Men tolerate depression less well than women, and are more likely to commit suicide (the commonest group for suicide are white males in their early seventies). It is one of the 'icebergs' of medicine: the majority of cases go unrecognized and therefore untreated.

Management of depression has improved considerably in the last few years with the introduction of medications that have less anticholinergic side effects and work more specifically on the main site that chemically produces the sense of depression: the serotonin reuptake system. The medications of choice for first-time use, and the most easily prescribable by the primary care clinician, are the selective serotonin reuptake inhibitors (SSRIs), such as fluoxetine, paroxetine and sertraline.[20]

The point of recognizing that depression is common is that a lack of libido is a symptom of depression. If there is truly anhedonia (a lack of interest in everything that was previously pleasurable, with the inability even to rise to the occasion when something good happens), then major depression is likely, and an antidepressant should be attempted. Table 4.3 summarizes the DSM-IV criteria for major depression. If these symptoms are sought and carefully addressed by primary care physicians, a great service will be done, because this treatable illness will be found and fixed more frequently.

Allowing depression to go untreated leaves the couple coping with a problem which will upset relationships, will decondition the patient, and may well lead to permanent sequela even though the depression itself generally eventually lifts. Suicide is always a risk if depression is untreated. Thus the aggressive discovery of depression and its enthusiastic management are an essential hallmark of good primary care practice.

Although most antidepressants have been associated with modifying sexual response in a negative way, if the lack of libido is clearly associated with depressive systems, it is likely that the sexual problem will respond to the antidepressant. However, separate sexual counseling may be required, since the sexual dysfunction may be persistent even when the depression has been treated and relieved.

PERSISTENT PROBLEMS

Despite all these simple measures described, and despite formal sexual therapy for those with psychological problems and primary sexual disorders, some cases will have persistent impotence or other persistent physical problems.

There are many physical techniques for overcoming neurogenic impotence or even psychogenic impotence when it affects the erectile dysfunction. Intracavernous injection of prostaglandin E1 has been used.[21] In addition, penile implants and prostheses, including prostheses that allow controlled erection, have been successful in situations with men with persistent problems.[22] In addition, tumescence devices are now approved by the FDA.[23] These are pressure devices that enable engorgement of the penis to be achieved, thus allowing a large erection. These are prescribable devices, and available without embarrassment from surgical suppliers. However, prior to their use, it would generally be advisable to seek urologic consultation in case of correctable issues.

The use of testosterone injections to improve potency, with its obvious placebo effect, is still not certain, although many authorities believe that these injections can be helpful in situations that diminish sexual drive in men.

SUMMARY

The gynecologist is a primary care physician and must be prepared, like all primary care physicians, to inquire at all possible and appropriate junctures about sexual activity, recognizing that underreporting of sexual problems leads to their underrecognition and undermanagement, and thus to a great deal of human suffering. Simple techniques can be used to prevent and treat many sexual problems. Clinicians need to introduce sexual issues into the interview especially when medications that might interfere with sexual functioning are prescribed, when illnesses occur which will have sexual implications, and when procedures have to be carried out which have sexual implications. A number of illnesses that do not immediately have sexual overtones do have sexual implications, particularly in relation to sexual positioning. Depression is an often-unrecognized illness that intertwines with sexual dysfunction and must be vigorously addressed by primary care physicians. The clinician who is going to be truly useful to the patient in trying to encourage continuing good sexual activity of satisfaction to both partners late into life will need a circle of referring individuals with whom he or she works regularly, including a certified sexual therapist, so that the range of interventions that may help with these distressing problems can be offered to all patients.

REFERENCES

1 Ham R. Sexuality. In: Ham R, Sloane P, ed. *Primary Care Geriatrics: A Case-Based Approach* St. Louis; Mosby YearBook, 1997.

2 Smith RW: Adult sexual behavior in 1989: Number of partners, frequency of intercourse and risk of AIDS. *Fam Plann Perspect* 3: 102, 1991.

3 Ehrhardt AA, Wasserheit, JN: Age, gender, and sexual risk behaviors for sexually transmitted diseases in the United States. In: Wasserheit SO *et al.*, eds. *Research Issues in Human Behavior and Sexually Transmitted Disease in the AIDS Era*. Washington, DC: American Geriatrics Society For Mocrobiology, 1991, p. 97.

4 Corbett L: The 1st sexual taboo: Sex in old age. *Med Aspects Hum Sexuality* 15: 117, 1981.

5 Masters WH, Johnson VE: Sex and the aging process. *J Am Geriatr Soc* 29: 385–390, 1981.

6 Masters WH, Johnson VE: *Human Sexual Response*. Boston: Little Brown, 1966.

7 Masters WH, Johnson VE, Kolodny RC: *Human Sexuality*. Boston: Little Brown, 1982.

8 Szasz G: Sexual incidents in an extended care unit for aged men. *J Am Geriatr Soc* 31: 407–411, 1983.

9 Wassow M, Loeb MB: Sexuality in nursing homes. *J Am Geriatr Soc* 27: 73–79, 1979.

10 Butler RN, Lewis MI: *Sex After 60: A Guide for Men and Women in Their Later Years*. New York: Harper & Row, 1976.

11 Renshaw D: Sex, age and values. *J Am Geriatr Soc* 33: 635–643, 1985.

12 Kass MJ: Sexual expression of the elderly in nursing homes. *Gerontologist* 18: 372–378, 1978.

13 McCartney JR *et al.*: Sexuality and the institutionalized elderly. *J Am Geriatr Soc* 35: 331–338, 1987.

14 Comfort A: Sexuality in the old. In: *Practice of Geriatric Psychiatry* New York: Elsevier North Holland, 1980.

15 Dhabuwala CB *et al.*: Myocardial infarction and its influence on male sexual function. *Arch Sex Behav* 15: 599, 1986.

16 McCoy NW *et al.*: Relationship among sexual behavior, hot flashes, and hormone levels in premenopausal women. *Arch Sex Behav* 14: 385, 1985.

17 Semmens JP *et al.*: Effects of estrogen on vaginal function in postmenopausal women. *JAMA* 248: 3445, 1982.

18 Drugs causing sexual dysfunction. *Med Lett* 34(876): 73–78, 1992.

19 Rowland KF, Haynes SN: A sexual enhancement program for elderly couples. *J Sex Marital Ther* 4: 91, 1978.

20 Lammers JE, Ham R: Depression and failure to thrive. In: Ham R, Sloane P, eds. *Primary Care Geriatrics: A Case-Based Approach*. St. Louis: Mosby YearBook, 1997.

21 Intracavernous injection of alprostadil for erectile dysfunction. *Med Lett* 37(958): 83–84, 1995.

22 Morely JE, Kaiser FE, Johnson LE: Male sexual function. In: Gassel CK *et al.*, eds: *Geriatric Medicine* 2nd edn. New York: Springer-Verlag, 1990.

23 Korenman SG *et al.*: Use of a vacuum tumescence device in the management of impotence. *J Am Geriatr Soc* 38: 217–220, 1990.

5

Contraception in perimenopause

SHAWKY ZA BADAWY

STEROIDAL ORAL CONTRACEPTIVES

Steroidal oral contraceptives were approved for use in the United States by the FDA in 1960. This followed a series of research work and clinical trials pioneered by Gregory Pincus and John Rock.[1] Their work constituted the foundation for a revolution in contraceptive technology.

The need for contraception in the perimenopausal years is important because of the high incidence of dysfunctional uterine bleeding due to anovulatory cycles and the high rate of termination of pregnancies during that stage of women's lives. Pregnancies above the age of 40 are associated with high maternal complications related to hypertension, diabetes and hemorrhages, and also maternal mortality. The estimated annual maternal deaths related to pregnancies in women above the age of 40 are about 42.9 per 100,000. Furthermore, the rate of termination of pregnancy is very high in women above the age of 40. It is estimated that the ratio is about 43.9 terminations per 100 pregnancies in this age-group. This is as high as termination of pregnancies in women below the age of 20. These termination rates are the highest of any other age-group in women.[2]

The use of contraception in general in the perimenopausal years is extremely low.[3] This is related to the fact that education in the use of contraception in this age-group is lacking. It is the duty of the primary care physician to counsel patients on the advantages and disadvantages of the use of contraception at this stage of their lives and to follow up on any side effects which might occur. Certainly, the use of steroidal oral contraceptives has many advantages for this age group, including contraceptive and noncontraceptive benefits.[4]

Since the early studies in the sixties, physicians and women have been concerned about side effects related to the pill. However, there have been many changes in the formulation of the pill to make it as effective as the parent pill but with significant reduction in side effects.

PHARMACOLOGY OF STEROIDAL ORAL CONTRACEPTIVES

Steroidal oral contraceptives are made up of a combination of an estrogen and a progestogen. The estrogen is ethinyl estradiol or mestranol. Ethinyl estradiol has an ethinyl group at the 17 position of the estradiol ring. The addition of this ethinyl group renders estradiol active orally. Mestranol has the same formula of ethinyl estradiol, but in addition it also has a methyl group attached to the three position. There has been a long debate about the efficacy of mestranol compared to ethinyl estradiol. This debate does not continue today because of the fact that mestranol has to be demethylated in the liver to be converted to ethinyl estradiol in order to be effective. Mestranol cannot attach itself to estrogen receptors. The biological efficacy, therefore, is not different from that of ethinyl estradiol. Furthermore, all the recent contraceptive pills on the market today have ethinyl estradiol as the estrogen component.[5]

The progestogen component of the steroidal oral contraceptive pill is a derivative of testosterone, which has been modified by removal of the 19-carbon from the parent compound and the addition of the ethinyl group at the 17 position. The removal of the 19-carbon from the compound changes the major hormonal effect from that of an androgen to that of a progestogen.[6,7] Accordingly, the progestational derivatives of testosterone are known as 19-nortestosterone. The 19-nortestosterone preparations are of two major groups. One group is the estranes, including norethindrone, norethynodrel and ethynodiol diacetate. The other group of progestogens is the gonanes, including levonorgestrel and the new generation of progestogens, mainly norgestimate, desogestrel and gestodene.[8]

Most of the progestogens related to norethindrone are converted to the parent compound for their effect on the various cellular structures. For the new generation of progestogens, some metabolic change has to occur to render them effective at the cellular level. Desogestrel is converted to 3-keto-desogestrel. Gestodene is converted into various progestational compounds, and norgestimate is metabolized to several compounds including 17-deacetilated norgestimate, 3-keto-norgestimate and levonorgestrel. The new generation of progestogens is very highly progestational. Their progestational activity is around eight to 20 times that of norethindrone. They have a high binding affinity to progesterone receptors and very minimal binding affinity to androgen receptors.

Because of the reduction of the dosage of estrogen and progestogen along the years to reduce side effects, and because of the introduction of the new generation of progestogens, the steroidal oral contraceptives have been classified into various generations. The first generation includes preparations containing more than 50 µg of ethinyl estradiol. This type of pill is no longer in use. The second-generation oral contraceptives are those containing 35 µg or less of ethinyl estradiol and a progestogen other than gestodene or desogestrel. Preparations containing norgestimate are included in the second-generation products. Third-generation oral contraceptives are defined as products containing low doses of ethinyl estradiol, usually 30 µg or less, and gestodene or desogestrel. Progestin-only pills are defined as those pills with a progestogen without any estrogen added. These are rarely used.[9, 10]

After the oral administration of the steroidal oral contraceptive, it is absorbed from the gastrointestinal tract. The estrogen and progestogen components reach a peak level within four to six hours and remain effective in the circulation for over 24 hours. They are metabolized in the liver by conjugation and excreted mainly in the urine. The hormonal effect with regard to contraception will be evident if the pill is used regularly on a daily basis.

INDICATIONS FOR USE OF STEROIDAL ORAL CONTRACEPTIVES IN PERIMENOPAUSE

Contraception

The birth control pill is the most effective method of contraception in general and especially in this age-group of women. It will protect perimenopausal women against unwanted pregnancies, prevent the high rate of termination of pregnancies, and prevent the high morbidity and mortality that accompany pregnancies at this age. The contraceptive effect is due to suppression of gonadotropins and ovulation, and changes in cervical mucus and the endometrium that lead to the antifertility effect.[11]

Treatment of dysfunctional uterine bleeding

Perimenopause is associated with a high incidence of dysfunctional uterine bleeding due to ovulatory dysfunction. Anovulation and oligo-ovulation are common phenomena due to marked reduction in the number of available follicles in the ovaries. Endometrial biopsies reveal the proliferative or hyperplastic effect of unopposed estrogen on the endometrium. To treat these cases and to prevent recurrence of such a problem, the use of birth control pills has been shown to be very effective. This will lead to secretory endometrium with atrophic changes. It will also lead to regular withdrawal bleeding and prevent the social inconveniences related to irregular bleeding. It will reduce the amount of bleeding per cycle and hence will increase the iron stores in the body and prevent the occurrence of hypochromic anemias.

NONCONTRACEPTIVE BENEFITS OF THE USE OF BIRTH CONTROL PILLS IN PERIMENOPAUSE

Prevention of epithelial ovarian cancer

It is known that pregnancy and breast-feeding are associated with reduction in the risk of occurrence of ovarian cancer. This is largely due to suppression of ovulation. Several studies support the role of suppression of ovulation in prevention of epithelial ovarian cancer. It has been shown that women using oral contraceptives have a 40% reduction in the risk of ovarian cancer compared with nonusers. This protection was found to last for ten years or more after one year of use of oral contraceptives. This protection rate could increase up to 80% with use of oral contraceptives for ten years or more.[12]

Protection against endometrial cancer

The world literature indeed supports the view that oral contraceptives significantly protect against endometrial cancer. The reduction rate is found to be 50% in oral contraceptive users with at least twelve months of use. This protection extends up to 15 years after discontinuation of the use of oral contraceptives. The protection against endometrial cancer was found to be related to adenocarcinoma, adenoacanthoma and adenosquamous carcinomas.[13]

Prevention of osteoporosis

Estrogen is known to be an important hormone in maintaining bone mass during reproductive years. This is supported by the findings of bone loss in amenorrhea, oligomenorrhea and irregular cycles in women. Furthermore, estrogen therapy has been shown to prevent bone loss in postmenopausal women.[14]

There have been several studies in premenopausal women to evaluate the use of oral contraceptives and their effect on bone mass. Some studies showed an increase in bone mass in users of oral contraceptives.[15,16] Others did not show such advantage.[17,18] More studies are needed to control for various factors as diet and exercise before reaching a conclusion.

OTHER CONSIDERATIONS FOR USE OF ORAL CONTRACEPTIVES

Cervical cancer

Some studies have reported an increased risk of cervical cancer and other studies have reported absence of risk with the use of oral contraceptives. These differences in the various studies are due to several factors, including sexually transmitted diseases, number of sexual partners and screening capabilities using the proper cytology procedures. In some studies controlling for all these confounding factors, investigators concluded that there was no increase in the incidence of cervical cancer with the use of the pill.[19,20]

A recent study by investigators and the World Health Organization addressed the relationship between the use of oral contraceptives and invasive adenocarcinomas and adenosquamous carcinomas of the uterine cervix. The study was prompted by the increase in the incidence of cervical adenocarcinomas in women under the age of 35 years betwen the early 1970s and mid 1980s. However, in recent years the incidence of adenocarcinomas and adenosquamous carcinomas of the uterine cervix has not been increasing and may have been decreasing.

This study found an increased risk of developing adenocarcinoma and adenosquamous carcinoma of the cervix with increase in parity, decrease in age of first intercourse, history of sexually transmitted diseases and low socioeconomic status. The risk of both histologic types of cervical carcinoma was lower in women with prior Pap smears, use of intrauterine devices and over 12 years of education. The relative risk of developing adenocarcinoma of the cervix was 1.6 and 1.1 for adenosquamous carcinoma of the cervix in oral contraceptive users. The relative risk decreased with the discontinuation of oral contraceptives. The relative risk also decreased with the use of low-progestogen types of oral contraceptives. Certainly, more studies are needed to address the effects of the recent low-dose pills on the incidence of such varieties of cervical cancer.[21,22]

Some other studies found that there was no increase in invasive disease; however, there was an increase in preinvasive disease. The presence of cervical dysplasias does not contraindicate the use of the birth control pill. However, this means that women on oral contraceptives should be screened regularly by proper Papanicolaou smears. Any evidence of dysplasia should be actively treated to prevent recurrence and progression.

Breast cancer

Several individual studies revealed discrepant results. The use of meta-analysis of various large numbers of studies revealed the absence of association between the use of oral contraceptives and the occurrence of breast cancer, with a relative risk of one. It is also to be noted that these results were based on oral contraceptives with high doses of estrogen. When studies were done disregarding the type of dose of hormones in these oral contraceptives, there was no association with the occurrence of breast cancer. When the analysis of the data was done for women using oral contraceptives below the age of 45, there was found to be a slight increase in the relative risk. It is also to be noted that there are many risk factors for the occurrence of breast carcinoma, including genetic predisposition due to family history, obesity and high-fat diet. All these factors have to be taken into consideration in analysis of any data.[23–25]

Metabolic effects of oral contraceptives

The use of the first generation of oral contraceptives was associated with changes in carbohydrate metabolism. Studies have shown increase in blood sugar levels as well as in insulin levels due to increased resistance to insulin at the peripheral tissues. With the use of low-dose formulations and use of the new progestogens, these changes are minimal or nonexistent.[26] Indeed, low-dose formulations can be given to patients who are prediabetic or diabetic.[27]

Effect on lipid metabolism

First-generation oral contraceptives have shown various changes in the lipid profile of women, depending on the dose of estrogen and the type of progestin which was present in the pill. With the use of the low-dose formulations and the new progestogens, these changes are minimal; their effect on women's health is not known.[28]

Liver tumors

Following the early use of oral contraceptives in the sixties, some reports described the rare occurrence of liver adenomas in women users. These adenomas were known to regress following discontinuation of pill use.[29] These were benign tumors and occurred in women using oral contraceptives with high estrogen and progestogen components. The patients usually present with upper-quadrant discomfort. Examination reveals liver enlargement, and the tumor is diagnosed by ultrasound or CT scan of the liver area. Liver biopsy confirms the diagnosis of a benign adenoma. There has been no reports regarding the occurrence of such tumors with the use of low-dose formulations.

The relationship between the use of oral contraceptives and the occurrence of liver cancer has been evaluated recently. There is a suggestion that estrogens and progestogens have a role in initiation and promotion of carcinogenesis in the liver. A population-based study from the United States, Sweden and Japan does not suggest any increased risk for liver cancer.[30]

Cardiovascular disease

The early studies with the first generation of oral contraceptives have shown increased incidence of cardiovascular disease in current oral contraceptive pill users.[31] With the use of the low-dose formulations, the incidence of myocardial infarction has been reduced.[32] Although some studies have shown some increase in risk, others revealed weak association.[33]

The risk of myocardial infarction among current oral contraceptive pill users is about three cases per million. Oral contraceptive pills multiply the effects of such risk factors as smoking, diabetes, hypertension and hyperlipidemia on the risk of myocardial infarction.[34]

The most recent studies regarding the use of low-dose birth control pills and their effect on the cardiovascular system revealed no increase in the risk of stroke, whether it is thrombotic or hemorrhagic.[35] However, the association between cardiovascular disease and smoking is very high.

Relationship between the use of oral contraceptives and the incidence of thromboembolism

Recently, there have been more publications regarding thromboembolism and its relation-ship to the use of oral contraceptives. This is not a new phenomenon. The use of oral contraceptives should be contraindicated in those patients who are more predisposed to these problems, such as patients with large varicose veins in the lower limbs, a history of venous thrombosis, thromboembolism, marked obesity and diabetes mellitus. The inci-dence of thromboembolism has been found to be related to the dose of estrogen. The higher the dose, the higher the incidence. With the use of low-dose formulations, it is well established by various studies that the incidence of thromboembolism has decreased. Recently, a multicenter, transnational research group study on oral contraceptives con-cluded that there is a slight increase in the risk of thromboembolism in patients using the third-generation progestogens; namely, gestodene, desogestrel and norgestimate. The study also found that the probability of death due to venous thromboembolism for women using these progestogens is about 20 per million users per year, compared to 14 per million users per year for second-generation progestogens and five per million per year for nonusers.[9] However, the same group found that there is a protective effect of the third-generation progestogens against myocardial infarction as compared to the second generation.[36]

The Food and Drug Administration (FDA) in the United States looked into this data and other analysis of the data by other United States centres, and concluded that there is no need for alarm. However, the FDA recommended that patients be counseled and felt there is no need to change patients who are comfortable with this type of oral contraceptive for another one unless the patient requests this change. (FDA-Talk paper T95–61, Rockville, MD, November 14, 1995).

CONCLUSION

The use of low-dose oral contraceptive pills in the perimenopausal years has many advantages. However, the treating physician should always project the most recent data to the patients with regards to side effects. When patients are aware of all these data, they will make an intelligent decision about their use and they will also comply with follow-up. The treating physician should follow up these patients every six months to a year with the regular general physical evaluation, including blood pressure measurements, breast evaluation, mammograms, pelvic examinations and Pap smears. Any side effects should be discussed and treated when necessary.

Due to the developments in oral contraceptive pills with regards to the new progestogens as well as low-dose formulations, it is the consensus and the clinical practice to prescribe low-dose formulations to all patients who are candidates for such a method of contraception. The new formulations with the low dosage have definitely led to marked reduction in side effects and have added to the advantages of oral contraceptives, especially for the perimenopausal patient. In 1989, after reviewing the relative risks and benefits of oral contraceptives, the Food and Drug Administration recommended that the upper age limit of 40 to be lifted for healthy, nonsmoking women. (FDA Advisory Committee on use of oral contraceptives in older women. On Line http: //www.fda.gov/bbs/topics/Answers/ANS00120.htmL, October 31, 1989). This has been a great breakthrough and has added a line of treatment which could be used effectively by physicians to prevent pregnancy and to correct irregular cycles due to oligo-ovulation in perimenopausal women. In spite of the marked research which has been going on to demonstrate the advantages and safety of oral contraceptives, women are still concerned about the use of the pill. This has been due to the fact that information given to them is not adequate and needs to be improved. The American College of Obstetricians and Gynecologists conducted a Gallup survey in 1985, repeated in 1993, to study the impressions and perceptions of women about oral contraceptives. (American College of Obstetricians and Gynecologists office of public information's poll shows women still sceptical of contraceptive safety. ACOG news release, January 1994). The proportion of women who believed there were substantial health risks associated with oral contraceptive use declined significantly from 76% in 1985 to 54% in 1993. However, 65% of women in 1993 still believed the pill was as hazardous as pregnancy. Only 20% volunteered that the pill helped regulate their menstrual cycles. The American Medical Association Harris Poll conducted another survey which focused on general reproductive health concerns, sexuality and contraception. Fifty-six percent of the respondents believed a woman should periodically give her body rest from oral contraceptive pills, and 50% thought the pill user needed to wait more than three months to attempt pregnancy after discontinuation of the pill. The Kaiser Family Foundation conducted another survey in January 1996 to study public perceptions about contraception. The result of that survey showed that 90% of reproductive-age women did not know the protective effect of the pill against osteoporosis and ovarian cancer, 33% considered the pill more likely to produce heart problems and only 25% considered the pill safe. The Association of Reproductive Health Professionals survey in January 1996 also revealed that many women are not aware of the noncontraceptive health benefits of oral contraceptives.

All these surveys suggest that physicians and other health professionals in the offices need to listen to the patients, answer their questions, alleviate their fears and document to them the data according to the most recent research studies. If this is done, the use of birth control pills in reproductive-age women as well as during perimenopause will be very much accepted, its advantages will be shown to be far superior to any side effects, and this will lead to better health achievements in these women.

INJECTABLE CONTRACEPTION: DEPOMEDROXYPROGESTERONE ACETATE (DMPA) (DEPO PROVERA)

DMPA has been in use for contraception for over 20 years in about 50 countries worldwide. In October 1992, the FDA approved its use in the US for contraception. The data from 11 studies during all these years has demonstrated that DMPA is safe as a contraceptive and that it has many other advantages. It has a very high contraceptive efficacy comparable to oral contraceptives. The contraceptive failure rate ranges from 0.0 to 0.7 per hundred women per year of use.[37,38] It is given in the form of intramuscular injection in a dose of 150 mg every three months. The first injection is given during the first five days of the menstrual cycle. This protocol eliminates the strict rule of daily administration associated with the use of oral contraceptive pills.

The contraceptive effect of DMPA is due to the suppression of LH peak and the prevention of ovulation. It also causes thickening of cervical mucus, which creates a barrier against sperm penetration. In addition, prolonged use leads to atrophic changes of the endometrium and eventually causes amenorrhea.

The World Health Organization collaborative study of neoplasia and steroid contraception did not find any increase in the relative risk of breast, ovarian and cervical cancer among users of DMPA. Furthermore, the study found a significant decrease in relative risk of endometrial cancer in users of DMPA.[39]

DMPA is suitable for use in women who are prone to develop anemia, since the amenorrhea produced by this contraceptive restores iron stores in the body. It is also suitable for use in women with hemoglobinopathies and seizure disorders.

It can certainly be used safely in perimenopausal women for its contraceptive and noncontraceptive benefits. One of the main problems that may limit its use in this age-group is the incidence of breakthrough bleeding that occurs during the first year of use in some patients. Perimenopausal patients with dysfunctional uterine bleeding should use oral contraceptive pills.

The effects on lipid metabolism and carbohydrate metabolism is favourable but needs more studies. DMPA leads to estrogen levels equivalent to those of early follicular phase of the cycle. The effect on bone metabolism needs further evaluation.

CONTRACEPTIVE IMPLANTS: NORPLANT (LEVONORGESTREL)

Norplant was approved for use as a contraceptive by the FDA in December 1990. Norplant is made up of six capsules (34 by 2.4 mm each). Each capsule contains 36 mg of the progestogen levonorgestrel. Six capsules are inserted under the skin of the medial aspect of the arm. The process of insertion and removal requires training and is done after infiltration of the skin with local anesthetic agent. Levonorgestrel is released at a rate of 85 μg per day.[40] The serum levels of levonorgestrel remain effective as a contraceptive for almost five years after insertion. The contraceptive efficacy is similar to oral contraceptives and DMPA. The pregnancy rate is about 0.8 per hundred women for the five years of use.[41]

Norplant produces its contraceptive effect through the suppression of LH peak and the prevention of ovulation, altering cervical mucus characteristics to render it impermeable to sperm and, in the long run, causing atrophic changes in the endometrium.

The early data regarding metabolic effects showed absence of lipid changes or blood sugar changes with the use of Norplant.[42]

The main problem is related to irregular uterine bleeding in some patients that may lead to discontinuation of its use.[43] Norplant is an effective method for use in perimenopausal women. In the presence of dysfunctional uterine bleeding, other contraceptives may be of value to the patient to control the bleeding.

BARRIER METHODS FOR CONTRACEPTION

There has been a renewed interest in the use of these methods during the past two decades. This is due to the increase in the incidence of sexually transmitted diseases and pelvic infections. Perimenopausal women should be counselled on the use of such methods when there is contraindication of the use of other methods and also if patients request a barrier method as their preference for their lifestyle. The failure rate of the diaphragm varies from two to 23 pregnancies per hundred women per year.[44] The cervical cap has a failure rate comparable to the diaphragm. The use of the female condom has been approved by FDA recently. The failure rate is about 15 per hundred women per year.[45] Since it is a relatively new method, more data are needed to assess its efficacy.

Failure rates depend on patient motivation, proper application and follow-up of the instructions for use of every method. The efficacy increases with the use of spermicides with the barrier method. There are three spermicides approved by FDA for use: menfegol, octoxynol, and nonoxynol 9. The majority of spermicide preparations contain nonoxynol 9. Nonoxynol 9 has antimicrobial activity against gonorrhea and chlamydia.[46] In addition, nonoxynol 9 has been shown to inactivate herpes virus and HIV virus *in vitro*.[46] The failure rate for spermicides has been found to be in the range of 21% to 22%. The combination of spermicides with a barrier method definitely decreases the failure rate.

Patients may not be able to use such methods if they are allergic to the device or unable to follow instructions for insertion and removal. The use of barriers and spermicides achieves both contraception and prevention of sexually transmitted diseases.

REFERENCES

1 Pincus G: *The Control of Fertility*, New York: Academic Press, 1965.
2 Mishell DR: Oral contraceptives for women in their 40s. *J Reprod Med* 35: 447, 1990.
3 Bachrach CA: Contraceptive practice among American women, 1973–1982. *Fam Plann Perspect* 16: 253, 1984.
4 Speroff L: In: Speroff L, Glass RH, Kase NG, eds. *Clinical Gynecologic Endocrinology and Infertility*, 'Steroid Contraception' 4th edn. Baltimore: The Williams & Wilkins Company, 1989, p. 461–498.
5 Goldzieher JW: Selected aspects of the pharmacokinetics and metabolism of ethinyl estrogens and their clinical implications. *Am J Obstet Gynecol* 163: 318, 1990.
6 Edgren RA, Sturtevant FM: Potencies of oral contraceptives. *Am J Obstet Gynecol* 1976, 125, 1029–1038.
7 Stanczyk FZ, Roy S: Metabolism of levonorgestrel, norethindrone, and structurally related contraceptive steroids. *Contraception* 42: 67, 1990.
8 Speroff L, DeCherney A: Evaluation of a new generation of oral contraceptives. *Obstet Gynecol* 81: 1034, 1993.
9 Spitzer WO, Lewis MA, Heinemann LAJ, Thorogood M, MacRae KD on behalf of Transnational Research Group on oral contraceptives and the health of young women: Third-generation oral

contraceptives and risk of venous thrombolic disorders: An international case control study. *BMJ* 312: 83, 1996.

10 Vessey MP, Lawless M, Yeates D, McPherson K: Progestogen-only oral contraception. Findings in a large prospective study with special reference to effectiveness. *Br J Fam Plann* 10: 117, 1985.

11 Letterie GS, Chow GE: Effect of missed pills on oral contraceptive effectiveness. *Obstet Gynecol* 79: 79, 1992.

12 The cancer and steroid hormone study of the CDC and NICHD: The reduction in the risk of ovarian cancer associated with oral contraceptive use. *N Engl J Med* 315: 650, 1987.

13 The cancer and steroid hormone study of the CDC and NICHD: Combination oral contraceptive use and the risk of endometrial cancer. *JAMA 257: 796, 1987.*

14 Armamento-Villareal R, Villareal DT, Avioli LV, Civitelli R: Estrogen status and heredity are major determinants of premenopausal bone loss. *J Clin Invest* 90: 2464, 1992.

15 Goldsmith NF, Johnston JO, Picetti G, Gracia C: Bone mineral in the radius and vertebral osteoporosis in an insured population. *J Bone J Surg* 55–A6: 1276, 1973.

16 Lindsay R, Tohme J, Kanders B: The effect of oral contraceptive use on vertebral bone mass in pre and postmenopausal women. *Contraception* 34, 333, 1986.

17 Hreshchyshyn MM, Hopkins A, Zylstra S, Anbar M: Associations of parity, breast feeding, and birth control pills with lumbar spine and femoral neck bone densities. *Am J Obstet Gynecol* 159: 318, 1988.

18 Lloyd T, Buchanan JR, Ursino JR, Myers C, Woodward G, Halbert DR: Long-term oral contraceptive use does not affect trabecular bone density. *Am J Obstet Gynecol* 160: 402, 1989.

19 Brinton LA: Oral contraceptives and cervical neoplasia. *Contraception* 43: 581, 1991.

20 Irwin KL, Rosero-Bixby L, Oberle MW, Lee NC, Whatley AS, Fortney JA, Bonhomme MG: Oral contraceptives and cervical cancer risk in Costa Rica: Detection bias or causal association? *JAMA* 259: 591, 1988.

21 Thomas DB, Ray RM, and The World Health Organization Collaborative Study of Neoplasia and Steroid Contraceptives: Oral contraceptives and invasive adenocarcinomas and adenosquamous carcinomas of the uterine cervix. *Am J Epidemiol* 144: 281, 1996.

22 Gramm IT, Macaluso M, Stalsberg H: Oral contraceptive use and the incidence of cervical intraepithelial neoplasia. *Am J Obstet Gynecol* 167: 40, 1992.

23 Cancer and steroid hormone study, CDC and NICHD: Oral contraceptive use and the risk of breast cancer. *N Engl J Med*, 315: 405, 1986.

24 Rushton L, Jones DR: Oral contraceptive use and breast cancer risk: A meta-analysis of variations with age at diagnosis, parity, and total duration of oral contraceptive use. *Br J Obstet Gynecol* 99: 239, 1992.

25 Murray P, Schlesselman JJ, Stadel BV, Shenghan L: Oral contraceptives and breast cancer risk in women with a family history of breast cancer. *Am J Obstet Gynecol* 73: 977, 1989.

26 Vander Vange N, Kloosterboer JH, Haspels AA: Effect of seven low-dose combined oral contraceptive preparations on carbohydrate metabolism. *Am J Obstet Gynecol* 156: 918, 1987.

27 Hannaford PC, Kay CR: Oral contraceptives and diabetes mellisus. *Br Med J* 299: 315, 1989.

28 Walling M: A multicenter efficacy and safety study of an oral contraceptive containing 150 microgram desogestrel and 30 microgram ethinyl estradiol. *Contraception* 46: 313, 1992.

29 Vessey MP, Kay CR, Baldwin JA, Clarke JA, McLeoad IB: Oral contraceptives and benign liver tumors. *Br Med J* April 23: 1064, 1977.

30 Waetjen LE, Grimes DA: Oral contraceptives and primary liver cancer: Temporal trends in three countries. *Obstet Gynecol* 88: 945, 1996.

31 Boyce J, Fawcett JW, and Noall EQP: Coronary thrombosis and conovid. *Lancet* 1: 111, 1963.

32 Meade TW, Greenberg G, Thompson SG: Progestogens and cardiovascular reactions associated with oral contraceptives and a comparison of the safety of 50 μg and 30 μg oestrogen preparation. *Br Med J* 1: 1157, 1980.

33 Sidney S, Petith DB, Quesenberry CP, Klatsky AL, Ziel HK, Wolf S: Myocardial infarction in users of low dose oral contraceptives. *Obstetrics and Gynecology* 88, 939–944, 1996.

34 Stadel BV: Oral contraceptives and cardiovascular disease. *N Engl J Med* 305: 612, 1981.

35 Stergachis A: Epidemiology of the noncontraceptive effects of oral contraceptives. *Am J Obstet Gynecol* 167: 1165, 1992.

36 Trussel J, Kost K: Contraceptive failure in the United States: A critical review of the literature. *Studies in Family Planning* 18: 237, 1987.

37 World Health Organization Task Force on long-acting systemic agents for fertility regulation: Special program of research, development, and research training in human reproduction. A multicentered phase III comparative clinical trial of depot-medroxyprogesterone acetate given three monthly doses of 100 mg. Or 150 mg. Contraceptive efficacy and side effects. *Contraception* 34: 223, 1986.

38 WHO Collaborative Study of Neoplasia and Steroid Contraceptives. Breast cancer. *Lancet* 338: 833, 1991. Endometrial cancer. *Int J Cancer* 49: 186, 1991. Epithelial ovarian cancer. *Int J Cancer* 49: 191, 1991. Squamous cervical cancer. *Contraception* 45: 299, 1992.

39 Robertson DN, Sivin L, Nash H, et al.: Release rates of levonorgestrel from silastic capsules, homogeneous rods, and covered rods in humans. *Contraception* 27: 483, 1983.

40 Diaz S, Pavez M, Miranda P, et al.: Long-term follow-up of women treated with Norplant implants. *Contraception* 35: 551, 1987.

41 Singh K, Viegas OAC, Loke DFM, et al.: Effect of Norplant implants on liver, lipid and carbohydrate metabolism. *Contraception* 45: 141, 1992.

42 Shoupe D, Mishell DR, Bopp BS, et al.: The significance of bleeding patterns in Norplant implant users. *Obstet Gynecol* 77: 256, 1991.

43 Trussel J, Hatcher RA, Cates W, et al.: Contraceptive failure in the United States. *Studies in Fam Plann* 21: 51, 1990.

44 Bounds W, Guillebaud J, Newman GB: Female condom (Femidom). A clinical study of its use, effectiveness, and patient acceptability. *Br J Fam Plan* 18: 36, 1992.

45 Singh B, Cutler JC, Utidjian HMD: Studies on the development of a vaginal preparation providing both prophylaxis against venereal disease and other genital infections and contraception and noncontraceptive preparations on treponema pallidum and neisseria gonorrhoeae. *Br J Vener Dis* 48: 57, 1972.

46 Hicks DR, Martin LS, Getchell JP, et al.: Inactivation of HTLV-III/LAV-infected cultures of normal human lymphocytes by nonoxynol-9 in vitro. *Lancet* ii: 1422, 1985.

6

Early detection and intervention of postmenopausal osteoporosis

FATMA A ALEEM

Menopause is a physiologic event that brings the physician and patient together. This physiologic milestone gives physicians the opportunity to enrol women in health maintenance and preventive care programs. Contrary to popular opinion, menopause is not a signal of impending decline. Rather, it is a signal for the perimenopausal and postmenopausal patient to start a good health program. Demographic studies of life expectancy for the twenty-first century reveal a change in longevity for women with a mean menopause age of 52.

In 1900, the life expectancy for a woman had reached only 49 years. By 1991, the average life expectancy for a woman had reached 78.9 years. Today, once a woman reaches 65, her life expectancy is 84 years, while a man who has reached 65 can expect to live until 80. It is estimated that roughly two-thirds of the population of the United States will live past 85, which will bring the pattern of life expectancy to a 'rectangular society'. This means that fewer women are dying during childhood or during childbearing, and are more likely to live out their maximum life expectancy.[1,2]

The 'baby boomers', who make up the largest generation in U.S. history, have a projected life span of 90 years. This means that baby-boomer women will spend almost half of their lives as climacteric and postmenopausal. These same women will experience significant physiological changes that will bring them to their physicians. Therefore menopause is a great opportunity to educate these women and to involve them in a preventive health care programme that addresses problems due to ovarian failure and aging, such as early detection of osteoporosis, cardiovascular disease, cancer and pre- and postmenopausal depression

Estrogen deficiency at menopause is associated with the accelerated phase of bone loss in women. Due to declining estrogen levels following menopause, bone resorption is increased dramatically. This increase in bone resorption will result in low bone mass and a deterioriation in bone microarchitecture, which represent osteoporosis. Therefore, post-menopausal osteoporosis will lead to enhanced bone fragility and an increased fracture risk.

EPIDEMIOLOGY AND CLINICAL ASPECT OF OSTEOPOROSIS

Osteoporosis is a common preventable disease that causes an absolute decrease in bone mass, rendering the bones susceptible to fracture even after minimal trauma. This disease is a considerable public health problem affecting 25 million Americans, 80% of whom are women. Osteoporosis results in 1.5 million fractures each year.[3] Osteoporosis-related fractures will develop in most postmenopausal women. Related fractures develop in locations with a high content of trabecular bone, such as the vertebral body, the femoral neck and radius. These fractures often restrict patient quality of life. The fractured hip, for example, can result in a 20% chance of mortality after one year, and as many as one-fourth of fracture hip survivors will be confined to long-term care facilities.[3] Direct and indirect costs of osteoporosis are estimated to be above 10 billion dollars per year in the United States alone. Since osteoporotic fracture incidence and severity increases with age,[4] in coming years, with an increase in the aging population, osteoporotic hip fractures and their severity[4] will lead to substantial societal and economic costs.

MECHANISM OF OSTEOPOROSIS

The physician must keep in mind that osteoporosis is a lifelong process reflecting the patient's risk factors: nutrition, hormonal levels in the reproductive years, levels of exercise and response to various medications. All of these elements, in addition to other factors, are detrimental to bone mass.

Peak bone mass

Bone mass increases rapidly during childhood and adolescence, and continues to increase throughout early adulthood until peak bone mass is generally attained by the age of 30. The attainment of normal peak bone mass is influenced by different factors, such as genetic potential, which appears to contribute significantly to limitation of bone mass and to osteoporosis later in life,[5,6] as well as by other environmental factors, such as exercise during active years, calcium and vitamin D intake and hormonal factors. Skeletal bone is influenced by hormones such as estrogens, progestins, androgens, thyroid and parathyroid hormones, calcitonin, glucocorticoid and growth hormones.[7]

Prolonged estrogen deficiency at menopause, physiological or surgical, and prolonged amenorrhea during reproductive life are accompanied by an accelerated phase of bone loss. This loss is due to a significant increase in bone resorption resulting from hyperactive osteoclasts. Parathyroid hormone exerts both inhibitory and stimulatory effects on osteoclast activity, which depends on the pattern of exposure. Chapuy and colleagues[8] reported that calcium and Vitamin D supplements reduce secondary hyperparathyroidism and lower the risks of fractures in elderly women. Lifestyle elements such as competitive exercise or sedentary lifestyles, especially during the developmental years, will result in bone loss. Smoking and moderate to excessive alcohol consumption will increase bone loss and result in a higher incidence of fracture.[9,10]

EARLY DIAGNOSIS OF OSTEOPOROSIS

Osteoporosis is a silent disease that causes an absolute decrease in bone mass, rendering the bone susceptible to fracture. Therefore early diagnosis of low bone mass through quantifying bone mineral density (BMD), followed by appropriate intervention, is very important in protecting the patient against further bone loss. It is established that low bone mass is predictive of future fractures. Bone loss accelerates significantly with the onset of menopause. However, low bone mass risk in women should be assessed long before menopause begins (perimenopausal period), especially in women with high-risk factors for osteoporosis. The factors should alert the physician to begin screening, diagnosis and early intervention therapy for osteoporosis.

Osteoporosis diagnostic techniques

Conventional radiography is not sensitive enough for diagnosing low bone mass; however, it is used to detect fractures. Several commercially available methods are widely used to measure bone mass. The following methods for quantifying BMD have been developed, permitting clinicians to diagnose early stages of osteoporosis, follow the course of the disease and assess the success of therapy:

SINGLE-PHOTON X-RAY ABSORPTIOMETRY (SPA)

This technique has been in use since the 1960s. The mechanism for measuring bone mass is achieved by the attenuation of a collimated photon beam from a radionuclide source (Iodine-125), which passes through the peripheral skeleton, such as the radius or calcaneus.[11] SPA measurements require a constant tissue path length, so the object is scanned in a water bath. Therefore, this technique is not convenient to measure BMD in lumbar spine or proximal femur.

DUAL-PHOTON ABSORPTIOMETRY (DPA)

In DPA, a gadolinium 153 source emits gamma photons at two different energy levels. This process can be used for bone mass measurements in the central skeleton (femur and spine), which are two skeletal sites particularly at risk for osteoporotic fracture in menopausal women. Although the use of DPA allows separation of bone from the soft tissue, the accuracy is not compromised, but some potential for error remains in older patients who show calcification of the aorta or other soft tissue over the spine, which will affect the results. Also, lumbar spine examination requires more time and shows poor resolutions compared with other methods.

DUAL-ENERGY X-RAY ABSORPTIOMETRY (DXA)

DXA uses a different level of energy from DPA. It uses X rays rather than nucleotides. This is the most precise of the other commonly used densitometry techniques. This process is more accurate in measuring BMD of the lumbar spine and proximal femur, and is safer due to its required short exposure – two to six minutes versus 20 to 40 minutes when using DPA. Additionally, a lower dose of radiation (1 to 3 mrem versus 5 mrem with DPA use)[12] is required. DXA measurements assess absolute bone mineral density g/cm^2. Due to these advantages, and enhanced precision and accuracy, DXA has become the 'gold standard' for

```
                                         SCAN:       1.33     04/08/97
                                         ANALYSIS: 1.33     04/08/97
```

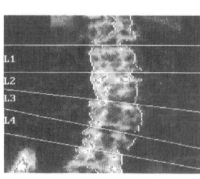

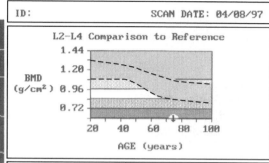

L2-L4 BMD (g/cm²)[1]		0.541 ± 0.01
L2-L4 % Young Adult[2]		45 ± 3
L2-L4 % Age Matched[3]		57 ± 3
L2-L4 sBMD (mg/cm²)[7]		515 ± 10

Age (years).........	75	Large Standard......	262.41	Scan Mode.......	Fast
Sex.................	Female	Medium Standard.....	197.13	Scan Type...........	DPX-L
Weight (lb).........	102.0	Small Standard......	139.05	Collimation (mm).....	1.68
Height (in).........	60	Low keV Air (cps)...	718265	Sample Size (mm).....	1.2x 1.2
Ethnic.............	Black	High keV Air (cps)..	429228	Current (uA)........	3000
System.............	7709	Rvalue (%Fat)....... 1.374(8.8)			

REGION	BMD[1] g/cm²	Young Adult[2] %	T	Age Matched[3] %	Z
L1	0.543	48	-4.89	62	-2.83
L2	0.628	52	-4.77	66	-2.74
L3	0.504	42	-5.80	53	-3.78
L4	0.479	40	-6.01	50	-3.99
L1-L2	0.588	51	-4.68	65	-2.64
L1-L3	0.557	48	-5.11	60	-3.07
L1-L4	0.542	46	-5.32	58	-3.29
L2-L3	0.563	47	-5.31	59	-3.29
L2-L4	0.541	45	-5.49	57	-3.47
L3-L4	0.494	41	-5.88	52	-3.86

Figure 6.1 *DEXA for lumbar vertebrae – original DXA print.*
[1] *Statistically 68% of repeat scans will fall within 1 SD.*
[2] *USA AP Spine Reference Population, Ages 20–45.*
[3] *Matched for Age, Weight (males 25–100kg; females 25–100kg), Ethnic.*
[7] *sBMD is standardized BMD. See J Bone Miner Res 1994; 9:1503–1514.*

bone densitometry. Figures 6.1 and 6.2 represent bone densitometry of lumbar spines and proximal femurs of two postmenopausal osteoporosis patients from our women's center.

QUANTITATIVE COMPUTED TOMOGRAPHY (OCT)

Quantitative computed tomography is the only method that provides a true volumetric (three-dimensional) measurement of bone density (g/cm³), and is the sole method that can estimate BMD separately in trabecular and cortical bone compartments. Although QCT can discriminate between osteoporotic and nonosteoporotic patients, its use is limited by higher expense and radiation dose compared to DXA. Following publication by Genant in

```
                                    SCAN:      1.33    04/08/97
                                    ANALYSIS:  1.33    04/08/97
```

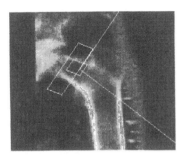

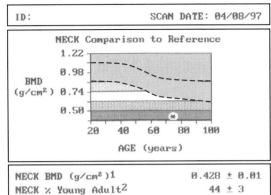

ID: SCAN DATE: 04/08/97

NECK Comparison to Reference

NECK BMD (g/cm²)1   0.428 ± 0.01
NECK % Young Adult2   44 ± 3
NECK % Age Matched3   55 ± 3

LUNAR®

Age (years).........	75	Large Standard......	262.41	Scan Mode.......		Fast
Sex................	Female	Medium Standard.....	197.13	Scan Type...........		DPX-L
Weight (lb)........	102.0	Small Standard......	139.05	Collimation (mm).....		1.68
Height (in)........	60	Low keV Air (cps)...	718265	Sample Size (mm).....		1.2x 1.2
Ethnic.............	Black	High keV Air (cps)..	429228	Region height (mm)...		60.0
System............	7709	Rvalue (%Fat).......	1.340(25.9)	Region width (mm)....		15.0
Side..............	Left	Current (uA)........	3000	Region angle (deg)...		62

```
NECK     : BMC⁵ (grams) = 1.79    AREA⁵ (cm²) =  4.2C
WARDS    : BMC⁵ (grams) = 0.54    AREA⁵ (cm²) =  1.96
TROCH    : BMC⁵ (grams) = 5.17    AREA⁵ (cm²) = 10.11
```

REGION	BMD[1] g/cm²	Young Adult[2] %	T	Age Matched[3] %	Z
NECK	0.428	44	-4.60	55	-2.89
WARDS	0.274	30	-4.89	43	-2.75
TROCH	0.511	65	-2.54	76	-1.46

Figure 6.2 *DEXA for proximal femur – original DXA print.*
[1] *Statistically 68% of repeat scans will fall within 1 SD.*
[2] *USA Femur Reference Population, Ages 20–45.*
[3] *Matched for Age, Weight (males 25–100kg; females 25–100kg), Ethnic.*
[5] *Results for research purposes, not clinical use.*

1982[13] on the use of QCT, most of us who were engaged in postmenopausal investigation and clinical management of osteoporosis used QCT until the development of the dual X-ray absorptiometry systems became available.

ULTRASONOGRAPHY

Ultrasonography was recently introduced for use in the detection of osteoporosis: the method applies bone ultrasound attenuation and speed of sound, and is expressed as meters per second. It is in its early development and not yet established for routine measurement of bone mass density.

BIOMECHANICAL BONE MARKERS

The determination of biochemical markers of bone turnover is a routine part of the diagnostic evaluation that rules out a number of metabolic bone diseases and assesses secondary causes of osteoporosis. Bone markers may represent resorption or formation; the most common markers are specific alkaline phosphatase, total alkaline phosphatase, percollagen I extension peptides and osteocalcin. However, most of these markers lack sensitivity and specificity. Resorption bone markers such as urinary calcium, hydroxy-proline, pyridinolene and dexoxy collagen Cross-links and related peptides, for example, N-terminal telepeptide are available as assays in certain laboratories. These assays are supposed to help identify accelerated bone loss as well as monitoring the effects of therapy.

Clinical application of bone densitometry: who should be monitored for osteoporosis?

Osteoporosis is most prevalent amongst older White and Asian women. Several epidemio-logic studies indicate that, as a group, women with osteoporosis tend to be of small build, live a sedentary lifestyle, have poor dietary calcium intake and are more likely to be smokers, consume more alcohol and coffee, and use certain types of medication such as glucocorticoids and antiepileptic drugs.

While these risk factors are fairly reliable in studying large groups of patients, they are unreliable for predicting the risks of fracture in postmenopausal patients.

Measurement of bone mass density is the only reliable means of diagnosing osteo-porosis; and measurement of bone mass provides the most reliable index for an individual at risk of sustaining an osteoporotic fracture.

In view of these considerations, there are three clinical applications for bone densitometry:

1 To establish a diagnosis of osteoporosis
2 To predict future fracture risk
3 To monitor changes in BMD due to medical problems or therapeutic intervention.

WORLD HEALTH ORGANIZATION DEFINITION OF OSTEOPOROSIS

The World Health Organization (WHO) recently defined osteoporosis in terms of BMD values: normal bone mass is designated as a value not lower than -1 SD from the mean BMD of a young adult value. Osteoporosis is defined as a BMD value lower than -2.5 SD from mean of BMD of young adults. Patients with BMD values in this range are at increased risk of fractures due to osteoporosis. Patients with values between 1 and 2.5 SD below average of young adults are said to have osteopenia and may be at increased risk of developing future osteoporosis. Johnson and colleagues[14] reported that a decrease of 1 SD in bone mass is associated with a 50% to 100% increase in fracture incidence.

PREVENTION AND THERAPEUTIC APPROACHES TO OSTEOPOROSIS

Estrogen replacement therapy (ERT)

Most menopause-related bone loss occurs during the first three to six years after the onset of menopause.[15] However, some bone loss due to low estrogen levels may continue for up to 20 years.[16] It was reported by Ettinger and colleagues[17] that early and long-term estrogen replacement therapy during menopause will significantly prevent and decrease bone loss and the incidence of osteporotic fractures.

Estrogen, the most common drug prescribed for older women, has become over the past decade the mainstay for osteoporosis treatment in the United States and much of Europe. Despite the support of researchers and epidemiologists, and its low cost, estrogen is rarely used in the prevention of osteoporosis. Only a small minority of postmenopausal women take estrogen long-term (over 10 to 15 years is needed to reduce fracture risk). Estrogen is generally used for one to two years, rather than long-term, to relieve postmenopausal symptoms. The reasons women reject estrogen therapy are complex, but include:

1   Fear of breast or endometrial cancer
2   Underestimation of risks from cardiovascular disease
3   Inconvenience of cyclical bleeding

Continuous combined therapy (estrogen and progestin) makes long-term therapy much more acceptable to patients.[18]

WHY, WHEN AND FOR HOW LONG SHOULD POSTMENOPAUSAL WOMEN BE ON ESTROGEN THERAPY?

Most gynecologists advocate prescribing estrogen at the time of menopause and continuing its therapeutic treatment over two to three years, which is expected to increase spine BMD by 5% and femur BMD by 2% to 3%, as reported by the PEPI trial.[19]

The optimum treatment is not known. When estrogen replacement therapy is discontinued, bone loss occurs at a rate similar to that following oophorectomy.[20] Cauley and colleagues[21] in 1995 studied a large number of women over 65 and assessed estrogen use and the incidence of fractures. Their results suggest that estrogen significantly reduces the risk of fracture if prescribed within five years of menopause and continued indefinitely.

Progestin administration is recommended during the last 12 to 14 days of the estrogen cycle to reduce the risk of endometrial hyperplasia; alternatively, it should be used at a small daily dosage continuously with estrogen.

Bisphosphonates

Bisphosphonates are analogues of inorganic pyrophosphates, which bind tightly to the bone's hydroxyapatite crystal matrix and reduce bone resorption by inhibiting osteoclast activity.

Among today's researchers, bisphosphonates are the preferred agents for treating osteoporosis, and their use has become routine clinical therapy for postmenopausal osteoporosis due to recent approval (November 1995) by the U.S. FDA. The currently most available bisphosphonate in the United States is alendronate (Fosamax from Merck), which is markedly more potent than its predecessor. Alendronate, with a recommended daily dose of 10 mg for osteoporosis therapy, inhibits bone resorption at doses at least 1,000 times lower than that inhibiting mineralization. With two identically designed, double-blind, placebo-controlled groups (aiming at six years; presenting three-year results), a study reported that postmenopausal women with osteoporosis had a mean BMD increase of 7% to 10% in the lumbar spin, 5% to 6% in the femoral neck and 7% to 8% in the trochanter, compared to placebo.[22]

The effect of Fosamax was tried on a fracture intervention study in postmenopausal women aged 55 to 81 using a placebo as control with low femoral neck BMD and an existing vertebral fracture. The study duration was 24 months and showed that alendronate was well tolerated and substantially reduced the frequency of morphometric and clinical vertebral fractures, as well as other clinical fractures.[23]

Another recent application of alendronate was in the prevention of osteoporosis when used early in menopause or in perimenopause in small doses.[24,25]

Calcium

In elderly women, the efficiency of calcium absorption is reduced. This diminished calcium will cause an increase in parathyroid hormone and subsequent bone turnover and bone loss.[25] It can be stated that during a woman's life it is essential to have adequate dietary calcium, which can provide the woman with adequate peak bone mass. However, this is not effective in preventing accelerated bone loss due to estrogen deficiency during the menopause years. Older women and those with osteoporosis require 1200mg to 1500mg calcium per day. Calcium carbonate is most efficient and economical.

Vitamin D

Administration of vitamin D in a dose of roughly 600 IU daily will benefit the patient with osteoporosis.

Calcitonin

Calcitonin is a peptide hormone secreted by parafollicular cells of the thyroid gland and is considered an antiresorption agent. Worldwide interest in calcitonin has declined as potent bisphosphonates have become available for clinical applications. The high cost and inconvenience of injectable calcitonin have led to infrequent use in many countries, except in Southern Europe and Japan. The new availability of salmon calcitonin in an intranasal formulation provides a more convenient alternative that may enhance clinical acceptance.

Fluoride

Over the past few years, there has been little clinical consideration of fluoride treatment of osteoporosis other than in Europe, where it is used. This is largely a consequence of negative findings in U.S. studies which were conducted using high doses of immediate-release sodium fluoride.

SUMMARY

Due to the significant impact osteoporosis has on a patient's life, we are faced with a strong sense of urgency and need for intervention. Safe and effective therapies are available for prevention and treatment of osteoporosis in postmenopausal women that can alter the course of this disease. However, most patients at risk for fractures are not being recognized and evaluated. Osteoporosis will continue to devastate the lives of millions of women in the U.S., especially with the increased life span of women, unless we take active measures in diagnosis, prevention and treatment of this disease. The climacteric period presents us with an opportunity to evaluate women and consider the appropriateness of measures to minimize the onset impact of osteoporosis in postmenopausal women who have already sustained an osteoporotic fracture. We currently have a myriad of treatment choices. Therefore it is never too early to prevent or too late to treat this disease.

REFERENCES

1 Olshansky SJ, Carnes BA, Cassel C: In search of Methuselah: Estimating the upper limits to human longevity. *Science* 1990; 250: 634.

2 Olshansky SJ, Carnes BA, Cassel C: The aging of the human species. *Scientific American* 1993; 4: 46–52.

3 Gamble CL: Osteoporosis: Making the diagnosis in patients at risk for fracture. *Geriatrics* 1995; 50: 24–33.

4 Edwards BJ, Perry HM III: Age-related osteoporosis. *Clin Geriatric Med* 1994; 10: 575–588.

5 Baner DC, Browner WS, Cauley JA, *et al.*: Factors associated with appendicular bone mass in older women. *Ann Intern Med* 1993; 118: 657–665.

6 Seeman E, Hopper JL, Bach LA, *et al.*: Reduced bone mass in daughters of women with osteoporosis. *N Engl J Med* 1989; 320: 554–558.

7 Lindsay R: Sex steroids in the pathogenesis and prevention of osteoporosis. In: Riggs BL, Meltron LJ III, eds. *Osteoporosis: Etiology, Diagnosis and Management.* New York: Raven Press, 1988; 333–358.

8 Chapuy MC, Arlot ME, Duboeuf F, *et al.*: Vitamin D and calcium to prevent hip fractures in elderly women. *N Engl J Med* 1992; 327: 1637–1642.

9 Baron JA, LeVecchia C, Levi F: The antiestrogenic effect of cigarette smoking in women. *Am J Obstet Gynecol* 1990; 162: 502–514.

10 Felson DT, Kiel DP, Anderson JJ, *et al.*: Alcohol consumption and hip fractures: The Framingham study. *Am J Epidemiol* 1988; 128: 1102–1110.

11 Cameron JR, Sorenson JA: Measurement of bone mineral in vivo: An improved method. *Science* 1963; 142: 230–232.

12 Jergas M, Genant HK: Current methods and recent advances in the diagnosis of osteoporosis. *Arthritis Rheum* 1993; 36: 1649–1662.

13 Genant HK, Cann CE, Ettinger B, Gordon GS: Quantitative computed tomography of vertebral spongiosa: A sensitive method for detecting early bone loss after oophorectomy. *Ann Int Med* 1982; 97: 699–705.

14 Johnston CC Jr, Slemenda CW, Melton LJ III: Clinical use of bone densitometry. *N Engl J Med* 1991; 324: 1105–1109.

15 Nordin BE, Need AG, Bridges A, Horowitz M: Relative contributions of years since menopause, age, and weight to vertebral density in postmenopausal women. *J Clin Endocrinol Metab* 1992; 74: 20–23.

16 Quigley ME, Martin PL, Burnier AM, Brooks P: Estrogen therapy arrests bone loss in elderly women. *Am J Obstet Gynecol* 1987; 156: 1516–1523.

17 Ettinger B, Genant HK, Cann CE: Long-term estrogen replacement therapy prevents bone loss and fractures. *Ann Intern Med* 1985; 102: 319–324.

18 Archer DF, Pickar JH, Bottinglioni F: Bleeding patterns in postmenopausal women taking continuous combined or sequential regimens of conjugated estrogens with medroxy progesterone acetate. *Obstet Gynecol* 1994; 83: 686–692.

19 Writing Group for the PEPI Trial: Effects of hormone therapy on bone mineral density: Results

from the postmenopausal estrogen/progestin intervention (PEPI trial). *JAMA* 1996; 276(17): 1389–1396.

20 Christiansen C, Christensen MS, Tranbol I: Bone mass in postmenopausal women after withdrawal of estrogen/gestagen replacement therapy. *Lancet* 1981; 1: 459–461.

21 Cauley JA, Seeley DG, Ensrud K, *et al.*: Estrogen replacement therapy and fractures in older women. *Ann Intern Med* 1995; 122: 9–16.

22 Chestnut CH III, McClung MR, Ensrud KE, *et al.*: Alendronate treatment of the postmenopausal osteoporotic women: Effect of multiple dosages on bone mass and bone remodeling. *Am J Med* 1995; 99: 144–152.

23 Denais Bach, *et al.* (Multiple study group): Randomised trial of effect of Alendronate on risk of fracture in women with existing vertebral fractures. *Lancet* 1996; 348: 1535–1541.

24 Bone HG, Downs RW Jr., Tucci JR, *et al.*: Dose-response relationships for alendronate treatment in osteoporotic elderly women – Alendronate Elderly Osteoporosis Study Centers. *J Clin Endocrinol Metab* 1997; 82: 265–274.

25 Sankaran SK: Osteoporosis prevention and treatment. Pharmacological management and treatment implications. *Drugs and Aging* 1996; 9: 472–477.

26 Riggs BL, Wahner HW, Dunn WL, Mazess RB, Oxford KP, Melton LJ: Differential changes in bone mineral density of the appendicular and axial skeleton with aging relationship to spinal osteoporosis. *J Clin Invest* 1981; 67: 328–335.

7

Perimenopausal breast disease

CHRISTINE M FINCK, MICHAEL M MEGUID

AND PATRICIA J NUMANN

INTRODUCTION

In nonsmoking women, menopause occurs around the age of 50, whereas smokers tend to become menopausal at an earlier age. Perimenopausal breast disease encompasses breast lesions arising in women between the ages of 40 and 70. The focus of this chapter will include those diseases occurring in the breasts of women during the perimenopausal period and include the following: fibroadenoma, fibrocystic disease and carcinoma. Knowledge of the anatomy and embryology of the breast is essential prior to exploring the associated pathology. A brief review is provided, and the reader is encouraged to consult the references for a more in-depth review.

NORMAL BREAST DEVELOPMENT[1,2,3]

The breast is a dermally derived organ that develops from a thickened portion of ectodermal tissue which forms a 'milk streak' coursing from pubis to axilla. Late in the first trimester, the milk streak atrophies, leaving only the pectoral portion which subsequently thickens into the nipple bud. The ductal system develops by invasion and downgrowth of primitive ectodermal cells from the nipple surface.

Anatomy of the breast and axillary space

In the mature breast, the parenchyma lies cushioned in fat between the layers of the superficial fascia of the pectoralis. Between the deep layer of superficial fascia and the pectoralis major muscle, the breast lays on loose areolar tissue – the retromammary space – and contains the lymphatics and small blood vessels. Deep to the pectoralis major muscle lies the pectoralis minor, and this muscle is enclosed in the clavipectoral fascia which extends laterally to fuse with the axillary fascia.

The axillary space is divided into three levels: 1) the external mammary, scapular, axillary vein, and central axillary groups, which lie lateral to the lateral border of the pectoralis minor muscle; 2) the central axillary group, which lies under the pectoralis minor muscle; and 3) the subclavicular nodes, which lie medial to the pectoralis minor muscle. At the apex of the axilla is the costoclavicular ligament (Halstead's ligament), at which point the axillary vein passes into the thorax and becomes the subclavian vein.

The lymphatics of the breast follow a centrifugal path from the subareolar plexus along major lactiferous ducts and then along efferent veins, and drain into peripheral nodes. The afferents lie under a deep layer of superficial fascia in the retromammary space. The major site of drainage is the central axillary node. More distal groups of drainage include the interpectoral Rottner's nodes, the subclavian nodes high along the axillary chain, and the supraclavicular nodes above the ipsilateral clavicle. Involvement of these distal nodes with tumor indicate advanced progression. In axillary dissection, intimate familiarity with the anatomic location of the nerves and their course is essential. The long thoracic nerve lies in the medial portion of the axilla along the chest wall. It innervates the serratus anterior muscle. Its accidental transection results in a 'winged scapula'.

Along the lateral border of the axilla lies the thoracodorsal nerve, which arises from the posterior cord of the brachial plexus and enters the axillary space under the axillary vein close to the entrance of the long thoracic nerve, and then crosses the axilla to the medial surface of the latissimus dorsi muscle. The lateral pectoral nerve innervates the lower third of the pectoralis major muscle, and preservation of this nerve prevents atrophy of this muscle. It follows a variable course, traveling, in the majority of patients, around the lateral margin of the pectoralis minor muscle. The sensory intercostal brachial and brachial cutaneous nerves supply sensation to the undersurface of the upper arm and skin of the chest wall, along the posterior margin of the axilla. Sacrifice of this nerve causes cutaneous anesthesia.

Each breast contains 15 to 25 independent glandular units called breast lobes. A single large duct, the lactiferous duct, drains each lobe via a separate opening on the surface of the nipple. The lactiferous ducts widen in the subareolar space to form lactiferous sinuses, which then exit through orifices on the nipple. The ducts are lined by low columnar/cuboidal epithelium, and the nipple surface is lined by squamous epithelium. The ducts branch and end blindly in clusters of spaces called terminal ductules/acini. A breast lobule consists of acini and small efferent ducts and ductules. The terminal ducts are invested in a specialized loose connective tissue that contains capillaries, lymphatics and other migratory mononuclear cells. The ductal system is surrounded by myoepithelial cells that have contractile properties and serve to propel the secretion of milk. Outside the epithelial and myopithelial layers, the breast is surrounded by a continuous basement membrane containing laminin, type IV collagen and proteoglycans. Invasion into this layer serves to differentiate *in situ* from invasive breast cancer.

BENIGN BREAST DISEASE[1,2,4]

Benign breast diseases are divided into three categories: nonproliferative, proliferative, and breast infections. Some studies have shown that the chances of developing benign breast changes are higher for women who have never had children, have irregular menstrual cycles, or have a family history of breast cancer. In addition, these benign breast conditions are more of a problem for women of childbearing age, whose breasts are more glandular.

Nonproliferative benign breast disease[1,4]

Nonproliferative benign breast conditions, in general, are not associated with an increased risk of developing breast cancer; they include the following;

SCLEROSING ADENOSIS

This is a benign condition involving an increased number of small terminal ductules or acini. This condition frequently causes breast pain. Calcifications indistinguishable from the microcalcifications of intraductal carcinoma are sometimes seen on mammograph, and often lead to breast biopsy. These lesions have no malignant potential. Other sclerosing lesions include radial scar and fat necrosis. Neither of these lesions has malignant potential; however, most require biopsy due to their confusing presentation on mammography, mimicking carcinoma.

CYSTS

These are epithelial-lined fluid-filled sacs that occur most often in women aged 35 to 50. These cysts are influenced by ovarian hormones, and can enlarge and become extremely tender just prior to menstruation. At least one woman in every 14 will develop a palpable cyst, and about half of these cysts will be bilateral. The formation of cysts appears to arise from destruction and dilation of lobules and terminal ductules. Cysts may occur as solitary abnormalities or gross breast cysts, or as a part of a generalized process of microscopic cyst formation. Diagnosis is made with physical examination and via cytological examination of specimens obtained by fine needle aspiration. Therapy consists of observation and fine needle aspiration of the cysts. Intracystic carcinoma is exceedingly rare. In addition, no studies demonstrate an increased risk of breast carcinoma in women with microscopic cysts. In patients with larger cysts, however, there remains some controversy. Most studies do not demonstrate a significant increase in cancers after long-term followup.

FIBROADENOMAS

These are benign tumors made up of structural and glandular tissue. On palpation, these masses are solid, round, mobile and painless, and have a rubbery consistency. Fibroadenomas are the most common type of tumor in women in their late teens and early twenties, but also present as late as the sixth decade of life. They occur twice as often in African–American women as in other American women. At operation, fibroadenomas will appear to be well-encapsulated and may easily detach from the surrounding breast tissue. These tumors may be distinguished from cysts through a fine needle aspiration, at which time no fluid is obtained. The risk of cancer in a newly discovered fibroadeonoma in a young woman is exceedingly rare. In women previously treated for fibroadenoma, the risk of breast cancer is about two times that of the general population. Treatment of a fibroadenoma ranges from observation to excisional biopsy.

INTRADUCTAL PAPILLOMAS

Solitary intraductal papillomas occur most commonly in women nearing menopause, whereas multiple papillomas are more common in younger patients. Papillomas usually produce a bloody discharge and may be associated with a breast lump. Solitary papillomas are true polyps of epithelial-lined breast ducts and are most commonly located under the areola. These lesions have no malignant potential. Multiple intraductal papillomas are more likely to be peripherally located and *are* associated with an increased malignant potential. They are diagnosed with a ductogram, and treatment consists of operative removal. These lesions can infarct, scar and develop squamous metaplasia, making pathological differentiation between invasive papillary carcinoma and a papilloma difficult.

Papillomatosis on the other hand, is not a true papilloma, but epithelial hyperplasia. It commonly occurs in younger women and is associated with fibrocystic change.

HAMARTOMA

This is a benign proliferation of variable amounts of epithelium and stromal supporting tissue. On physical examination, mammography and gross pathological inspection, a hamartoma is indistinguishable from the fibroadenoma. Curative treatment of a hamartoma includes surgical removal.

Proliferative benign breast disease[1,4–6]

Proliferative breast lesions are associated with an increased risk of developing breast cancer and include the following.

ATYPICAL DUCTAL HYPERPLASIA

This condition is thought to precede the development of ductal carcinoma *in situ* (DCIS). The rate at which atypical ductal hyperplasia may progress to either DCIS or invasive ductal carcinoma is unknown. This lesion is associated with about a 4.3–fold increase in the risk of developing breast cancer.

ATYPICAL LOBULAR HYPERPLASIA

This lesion is also associated with about a 4.3-fold increased risk of developing breast cancer.

Breast infections[1,4,7]

MASTITIS

This term describes a generalized cellulitis of breast tissue that may involve a large area of the breast but may not form an abscess. The pathophysiology appears to be an ascending infection beginning in the subareolar ducts and extending peripherally from the nipple. Clinical features include induration, erythema and pain. These lesions often respond poorly to antibiotics. Although mastitis may resolve spontaneously, more often, incision and drainage with appropriate use of antibiotics facilitates resolution. It is important to follow these patients to ensure complete resolution of symptoms. If the symptoms do not resolve, the possibility of inflammatory carcinoma needs to be ruled out.

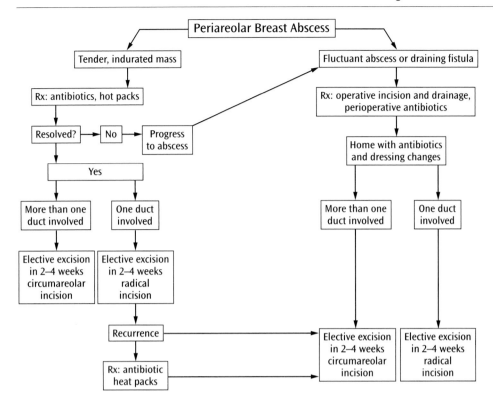

Figure 7.1 *Algorithm for the surgical management of breast abscesses based upon the stage of the disease.*

MAMMARY DUCT ECTASIA

This inflammatory condition causes distortion and dilation of the subareolar lactiferous sinuses. Treatment consists of antibiotics and surgical resection of the diseased mammary ducts. This condition commonly affects women nearing menopause.

PERIAREOLAR BREAST ABSCESS

Periareolar breast abscess includes a spectrum of clinicopathological events ranging from mammary duct ectasia and periductal inflammation/mastitis to subareolar induration, to the progressive evolution of later stages of the disease process presenting as a subareolar breast abscess, its repeated recurrences, and its subsequent related periareolar fistula. The disease is benign, most often originates in the large subareolar mammary collecting ducts and may manifest itself as a secondary inflammatory reaction. It is strongly associated with cigarette smoking. Treatment is based on the pathophysiology of the disease process and includes removal of the involved ducts. Meguid and colleagues have developed an algorithm for the surgical management of breast abscesses based upon the stage of the disease (Figure 7.1). Antibiotics used include a penicillin derivative and metronidazole. If patients are allergic to penicillin, clindamycin, erythromycin or cephradine may be substituted.

MALIGNANT BREAST DISEASES[1,2,8]

Breast cancer is the leading cancer in women and is second only to lung carcinoma in mortality. The incidence of breast cancer has been increasing steadily at 1% per year for the past 50 years and currently, a woman's lifetime risk of developing breast cancer is one in eight. Despite earlier detection, survival rates have not changed over the years.

Malignant breast diseases are broadly classified into epithelial tumors of cells lining ducts and lobules, and nonepithelial malignancies of the supporting stroma. In addition, tumors are further classified into noninvasive if they do not invade the basement membrane, and invasive if they penetrate the basement membrane.

DUCTAL CARCINOMA *IN SITU* (DCIS)

This is a benign lesion in which breast ducts become swollen with proliferating malignant epithelium. Pure intraductal carcinoma denotes a lesion that has no detectable invasion of the basement membrane. Histologically, the center of the lesion undergoes necrosis and the intraductal spaces fill with necrotic cellular debris. The central detritus may then undergo dystrophic calcification, producing even linear and branching calcification patterns that are picked up on mammography. In addition, DCIS may produce a palpable mass that is recognized on physical examination.

The subtypes of DCIS are solid or comedo type and papillary or cribriform. In the solid/comedo type, cells are closely packed within the ductal spaces. This type is more virulent and occurs more commonly. In the papillary/cribriform type, there are papillary projections of tumor cells into the ductal lumen with the presence of a branching, cribriform pattern filling the ducts. These types are less likely to calcify and less likely to produce a palpable mass.

Treatment and prognosis for patients with intraductal disease depends on variables such as multifocality, multicentricity and extent of the disease. It is important to note that DCIS may coexist with infiltrating ductal carcinoma.

LOBULAR CARCINOMA *IN SITU* (LCIS)

This is a benign breast disease characterized by a proliferation of small round epithelial cells within the lumen of multiple breast acini. It is quite uncommon for LCIS to form a palpable mass, and therefore it is not recognized on physical examination. It also does not produce any mammographic changes and is usually diagnosed incidentally.

INFILTRATING DUCTAL CARCINOMA

This is the most common malignant tumor of the breast. It arises from ductal epithelium and is invasive in nature, with infiltration into a variable amount of stroma as cords of malignant epithelium. Infiltrating ductal carcinoma is usually diagnosed after more distinctive breast disease have been eliminated. There is an *in situ* component to this tumor. A stromal reaction to the tumor may be intense, and at one time infiltrating ductal carcinoma was referred to as scirrhous carcinoma of the breast.

Clinically, most infiltrating carcinomas present as a mammographic abnormality or as a palpable mass. Microcalcifications are commonly found in the necrotic centers of the intraductal component. Important parameters to evaluate when dealing with breast cancers are tumor size, status of surgical margin, content of estrogen and progesterone receptors, and vascular invasion. In addition, nuclear and histologic grade, DNA content and estimation of the proliferating fraction (S phase) are often reported.

INVASIVE LOBULAR CARCINOMA

This form of breast cancer arises from the breast lobule and constitutes between 3% and 15% of all invasive breast cancers. Histologically, the tumor is composed of small round cells that infiltrate the surrounding stromal tissue in an Indian-file fashion. Invasive lobular carcinoma may present with a palpable mass, but does not have any distinguishing mammographic features. There appears to be a higher incidence of bilateral cancer or a second primary cancer in the contralateral breast in invasive lobular carcinoma.

OTHER BREAST CANCERS

These constitute all morphologic variants of common ductal carcinoma. In general, these cancers are less common and have a better prognosis than ductal carcinoma.

Medullary carcinoma of the breast is characterized by bizarre and anaplastic tumor cells surrounded by a lymphocytic infiltrate with a scant fibrous stroma.

Mucinous or colloid carcinoma of the breast is characterized by well-differentiated epithlial cells surrounded by a large accumulation of extracellular and extraluminal mucin that is secreted by the tumor cells. This tumor is less likely to metastasize than infiltrating carcinoma.

Tubular carcinoma is characterized by infiltrating tubular structures, lined by one cell layer with an open central space and a decreased propensity to metastisize.

It is important to note that each of the above tumors may coexist with common type of infiltrating carcinoma.

Staging of breast cancer[1,8]

Staging of breast cancer has evolved from the classifications proposed by the International Union Against Cancer (UICC) and the American Joint Committee on Cancer (AJCC). Staging is utilized to determine prognosis of patients after treatment and to allow for comparison of results within and between clinical trials.

Classification of breast cancer begins with evaluating the tumor (T), the nodal status (N), and for the presence of metastasis (M) as summarized in Table 7.1.

Risk factors[1,2,9–17]

Known risk factors may account for more than 40% of US breast cancer diagnoses, whereas 70% of patients who develop breast cancer will not have identifiable risk factors. Risk factors have been divided into age, gender, family history, ovulatory cycle and other factors.

AGE

In general, the incidence of breast cancer increases with increasing age. Breast cancer is exceedingly rare in patients younger than 20, and women under the age of 30 constitute less than 2% of total cases. In the eighth decade of life, the annual incidence rises to 300 cases per 100,000. Therefore, age is an important risk factor.

GENDER

Although males are at risk for developing breast cancer, the incidence is less than 1% of the incidence in females.

Table 7.1 *Breast Cancer Staging – TNM*

Tumor (T)

TX – a primary tumor that cannot be assessed
T0 – no evidence of a primary tumor
Tis – carcinoma *in situ*: intraductal carcinoma, lobular carcinoma *in situ*, or Paget's disease of the nipple with no tumor
T1 – tumor 2 cm or less in greatest dimension
    T1a – tumor less than 0.5 cm
    T1b – tumor more than 0.5 cm, but not more than 1 cm in greatest dimension
    T1c – tumor more than 1 cm, but not more than 2 cm in greatest dimension
T2 – tumor more than 2 cm, but not more than 5 cm in greatest dimension
T3 – tumor more than 5 cm in greatest dimension
T4 – tumor of any size with direct extension to chest wall of skin
    T4a – extension to chest wall
    T4b – Edema (peau d'orange) or ulceration of the skin of breast or satellite skin nodules confined to same breast
    T4c – both T4a and T4b
    T4d – inflammatory carcinoma

Nodes

NX – regional lymph nodes cannot be assessed
N0 – no regional lymph node metastasis
N1 – metastasis to movable ipsilateral axillary lymph nodes
    N1a – only micrometastasis with none larger than 0.2 cm
    N1b – metastasis to lymph nodes, any larger than 0.2 cm
        N1bi – metastasis to 1–3 lymph nodes, any more than 0.2 cm and all less than 2 cm in greatest dimension
        N1bii – metastasis to 4 or more lymph nodes, any more than 0.2 cm and all less than 2 cm in greatest dimension
        N1biii – extension of tumor beyond capsule of a lymph node metastasis less than 2 cm in greatest dimension
        N1iv – metastasis to a lymph node 2 cm or more in greatest dimension
N2 – metastasis to ipsilateral axillary lymph nodes that are fixed to one another or to other structures
N3 – metastasis to ipsilateral internal mammary lymph nodes

Metastasis

Mx – presence of distant metastasis cannot be assessed
M0 – no distant metastasis
M1 – distant metastasis (includes metastasis to ipsilateral supraclavicular lymph nodes)

GENETICS

Some 9.1% of breast cancers are attributable to having a family history of breast cancer. The risk of developing breast cancer in a woman whose mother or sister had the disease is 1.5 to 3 times that of the general population. Bilateral premenopausal breast disease in a relative has been associated with the highest risk of breast cancer development.

In 1990, Marie-Clare King mapped the first breast cancer susceptibility gene (BRCA1) to chromosome 17q21, and Mark Scolnick is credited with sequencing this gene. The BRCA1 gene confers an 83% risk of developing breast cancer and a 63% risk of developing ovarian cancer by the age of 70. The BRCA2 gene has also been recently mapped to chromosome 13q12, and it appears to confer the same risks of breast cancer as the BRCA1 gene. Several oncogenes and tumor suppressor genes have also been implicated in sporadic noninherited cases of breast cancer. Therefore, genetic testing will most likely play a greater role in the screening for breast cancer in the future and in the determination of treatment options.

OVULATORY CYCLE

Nulliparous women have a risk factor of 1.4 compared with multiparous women for the development of breast cancer. In addition, a decreased risk of breast cancer development has been found in women who become menopausal before the age of 40 and in women who have an oopherectomy before the age of 50. Women whose first pregnancy occurs after the age of 30 have a two- to five-fold increased risk of developing breast cancer compared with women who give birth before the age of 18. Also, approximately 3% of breast cancers are associated with pregnancy or lactation, and no studies have demonstrated a therapeutic role for abortion in altering the natural history of the disease. Biopsy and mastectomy can be well tolerated by the mother and fetus with the risk of spontaneous abortion following general anesthesia in the first trimester being approximately 1%.

The use of exogenous hormones in relation to the development of breast cancer remains controversial. The Center for Disease Control's Cancer and Steroid Hormone Study failed to find any increase in risk related to duration of oral contraceptive use or in users with a family history of breast cancer or a personal history of benign breast disease. On the other hand, there are several studies claiming that oral contraceptive pills (OCP) increase the risk of breast cancer. Brinton and colleagues reported in 1995 that the OCP increased the risk of breast cancer in women under age 35 who used the pill for six months or more. Compared to nonusers, these women had a 70% increased risk of developing breast cancer, and this risk was further increased among women who used the pill long-term, especially if they also began to take the pill before age 18. In addition, researchers at the Fred Hutchinson Cancer Research Center reported a 50% increased risk associated with taking OCP containing high amounts of progestin for at least one year under the age of 35. Also, the US Cancer and Steroid Hormone Study found that women of 20 to 34 who had ever used the pill had a 40% increased risk of breast cancer.

The use of postmenopausal hormone replacement therapy is also controversial and may be associated with a small increase in breast cancer risk in the range of 1.5 to 2.0 for moderate-dose conjugated estrogen therapy lasting for 10 to 20 years. Therefore, the benefits of hormone replacement therapy need to be balanced against the potential for developing breast cancer.

OTHER RISK FACTORS

There have been numerous reports of other factors contributing to or preventing the development of breast cancer, as follows.

Income
Some 18.9% of patients with breast cancer have a moderate or high income.

Exercise
Bernstein and colleagues in California found that regular and moderate exercise decreased a woman's risk of developing breast cancer by more than 60%.

Diet

Japanese-born women have a lower incidence of breast cancer compared with American-born Japanese women or Japanese women emigrating to the United States. This implies that diet plays a role in the development of breast cancer.

Alcohol

This has been found to be associated with an increased risk of developing breast cancer. The American Cancer Society has found that there is no increased risk of developing breast cancer for occasional users of alcohol, but the risk was elevated in women who consume heavy amounts of alcohol.

Screening for breast cancer[8,18-21]

During the 1990s, approximately two million new cases of breast cancer and 500,000 deaths from the disease are anticipated. As yet, there are no effective preventitive measures. Screening, the centrepiece of early detection, consists of breast self-examination, physical examination by a health professional and mammography. Only self-breast examination and mammography are discussed further, physical examination by a health professional being self-evident.

BREAST SELF-EXAMINATION

Formal monthly breast self-examination (BSE) after the age of 30 and within a few days after the menstrual period has been promoted as a method of early detection of breast cancer. However, no randomized study has produced data on the effectiveness of BSE in reducing mortality from breast cancer. One cohort study did find fewer deaths due to breast cancer and improved estimated five-year survival rates among women who reported performing BSE compared with women who reported no BSE. Also, it is important to note that 10% of all palpable breast cancers are not visible on mammogram and therefore, the importance of BSE becomes apparent, and all clinically suspicious palpable lesions should be biopsied.

MAMMOGRAPHY

Screening mammography has proved to be effective in reducing the mortality rate for breast cancer. The basic abnormalities assessed by radiologists interpreting mammograms are masses and calcifications. Other more subtle signs include architectural distortion, parenchymal asymmetry and neodensity in the breast. Lesions suspicious for malignancy include masses with inhomogenous density, irregular shape, and spiculated borders and calcifications with linear branching patterns, high spatial density, microcalcifications or many calcifications. The sensitivity of mammography has been reported to range between 85% and 90%. It has been suggested that sensitivity of mammography is lower by 10% for women between 40 and 49 because of the high density of the breasts. However, a study conducted by Davies and colleagues has demonstrated that in patients requiring breast biopsy, contemporary mammography is similar in accuracy in the younger patient when compared to the older, postmenopausal patient.

The accuracy of mammographic interpretation has been questioned. Despite the proven value of mammography in screening for breast cancer, its efficacy depends on radiologists' interpretations. In a study by Elmore and colleagues the diagnostic consistency between pairs of radiologists was 78%, and a substantial disagreement in management recommendations was noted. Therefore, while it is important to utilize mammography as a screening method, the limitations of this test must be kept in mind.

WHO SHOULD UNDERGO SCREENING?[8,21]

In women aged 40 to 49 years of age, there have been no randomized trials demonstrating a reduction in breast cancer mortality with five to seven years of follow-up. In the HIP study, a marginal reduction in mortality at 10 to 12 years was noted, but it is questionable whether this is statistically significant. Therefore, the National Cancer Institute's current recommendation is to consult a health care professional to discuss the advisability of mammography, taking into account family history of breast cancer and other risk factors. The NCI recommends annual clinical breast examination in this group.

In women aged 50 to 69, there is strong evidence that screening mammography on a regular basis is efficacious in reducing breast cancer mortality by 30%. The National Cancer Institute recommends women be screened every one to two years with a mammogram and an annual clinical breast examination.

In women over 70 years of age, there is not sufficient information in the randomized trials to evaluate. The NCI, however, recommends that these women should be screened unless otherwise indicated by health status.

OTHER DIAGNOSTIC PROCEDURES[2,22,23]

Ultrasound

Ultrasound is useful in the diagnosis of cystic disease and in the demonstration of solid abnormalities with specific echogenic features. The resolution of ultrasound is inferior to high-resolution mammography, and lesions less than or equal to 1 cm in diameter, unless cystic, will not be detected.

Fine needle aspiration (FNA)

FNA has become a routine part of the physical diagnosis of breast masses. In general, it is useful in differentiating solid from cystic masses. A formal open biopsy should be done if the needle aspiration produces no cyst fluid, or the cyst fluid is thick and blood-tinged, or the mass fails to resolve even though fluid is produced, or the mass reappears in the same area after more than two aspirations. The use of cytologic examination of aspirated material from a solid mass is helpful when a negative result is obtained, further work up, including an excisional biopsy, should be pursued. When a positive result is yielded, plans for treatment can be made with the patient.

Stereotactic core needle biopsy

There is evidence to suggest that stereotactic core biopsy is as accurate as needle localization and open surgical biopsy for nonpalpable breast lesions discovered with mammography. In a series of 300 consecutive stereotactic core needle biopsies, the sensitivity was found to be 100% with a 98% specificity. Using screen images, biopsy coordinates are calculated by a computer and a 14-gauge core needle is inserted into the breast, with stereotactic images confirming pre- and postfire localization. Specimen roentgenograms are then performed to evaluate for the presence of calcifications. This procedure can be done in an outpatient setting, causes minimal discomfort and morbidity, and can biopsy lesions as small as 3 to 4 mm.

Lymphatic mapping and sentinel node biopsy

For most tumors, the most predictive prognostic factor is the status of the regional lymph nodes. In breast cancer, the presence of regional metastases decreases five-year survival by approximately 28% to 40%. Currently, management of the axilla in a patient with breast cancer is controversial. Lymphatic mapping demonstrates the lymphatic drainage pattern from primary tumors and maps the drainage to regional lymph nodes. The first node in the basin is the sentinel lymph node (SLN) and is the presumptive initial site of metastatic disease. The histologic characteristics of the SLN reflect the histologic characteristics of the rest of the nodes in the basin, and should increase the sensitivity of routine histologic examination and allow for improved detection of micrometastases. In a study of 62 patients, the sensitivity of lymphatic mapping and SLN biopsy was 100%. The ideal procedure involves both vital blue dye mapping and radiocolloid mapping during axillary dissection. These two techniques are complementary and when used together, optimal results are obtained.

Operative therapy for breast cancer[1,8,24]

Surgery, as local therapy, remains the single most effective tool in the treatment of breast cancer. The introduction of mastectomy in the 1930s led to dramatic decreases in the death rate from breast cancer. Now, despite more than 30 years of prospective trials, there has been no substantial reduction in age-specific death rate.

Invasive breast cancers

Breast conservation with lumpectomy, axillary dissection and radiation therapy is equivalent in outcome to modified radical mastectomy for the therapy of most breast cancers.

Breast conservation[8,25]

Prospective randomized trials have demonstrated equivalent survival at five and 10 years between breast conservation treatment and modified radical mastectomy. The addition of radiation therapy to breast conservation therapy has reduced the local failure rate from 30% to between 5% and 7%.

There are certain standards for conservative breast treatment. Lumpectomy margins must be free of invasive carcinoma or DCIS for a margin of greater than one-fifth the size of the lesion. The overlying skin must be removed if the lesion is within 1 cm of skin or tethered to the skin in any way on preoperative physical examination.

The relative contraindications to lumpectomy include multifocal invasive carcinoma, multifocal DCIS, multiple high-risk lesions that increase the likelihood of an ipsilateral new breast cancer, inability of mammography to detect the original primary tumor, patients with tumors large relative to the size of their breasts, or breasts that are difficult to evaluate by physical examination and mammography.

The extent of axillary dissection varies between institutions. At Johns Hopkins, axillary dissection for breast conservation is defined as a generous axillary sampling to encompass over two-thirds of level 1 and 2 nodes in clinically node-negative patients. In clinically node-positive patients, a traditional full axillary clearance is performed. Radiation therapy to the axilla is reserved for those patients with more than five or six positive lymph nodes, bulky positive nodal disease or soft tissue extension in the axilla. Chemotherapy is associated with decreased recurrence in the axilla more often than radiation therapy.

Radiation therapy for breast conservation is typically given to the breast mound with doses of more than 5000 rad or 50 Gy.

Follow-up for breast-conserved patients includes mammograms of the conserved breast at six-month intervals for the first five years and annually therafter. A mammogram is taken of the opposite breast six months after the original therapy and then annually thereafter.

Modified radical mastectomy (MRM)[8]

In current practice the MRM includes near-total removal of breast tissue of the breast mound and axillary tail of Spence and an axillary sampling without complete axillary dissection. In complete axillary dissection, the incidence of lymphedema can reach 30%. In limited axillary dissection, on the other hand, the incidence of lymphedema is less than 5%, with no evidence of increased clinical axillary failure.

Several principles are advocated at Johns Hopkins when performing MRM in order to facilitate postmastectomy reconstruction. They include the following: complete excision of any biopsy scar; removal of the nipple in continuity with the major retroareolar ductal complex; removal of any skin tethered to the lesion or directly overlying a lesion within 2 cm of the skin surface; removal of all breast tissue from Camper's fascia to pectoralis major fascia with extension of the dissection to include the full axillary tail of Spence; and use of a skin-sparing incision when possible.

MANAGEMENT OF HIGH-RISK LESIONS[8,26]

The treatment of high-risk breast lesions such as ductal carcinoma *in situ*, lobular carcinoma *in situ*, and atypical ductal hyperplasia remains controversial. In DCIS, studies have shown that a recurrence risk of 1% to 5% per year in the ipsilateral breast each year after the diagnosis has been confirmed. Fifty per cent of recurrences are invasive ductal carcinomas, with approximately 30% of these metastatic to lymph nodes. Treatment ranges from confirmatory biopsy to lumpectomy, to prophylactic mastectomy. Thirty per cent of DCIS patients have multifocal lesions, and the NSABP B-17 study demonstrated a substantial risk of local failure after lumpectomy alone. The addition of radiation decreases this recurrence rate to 15% per year. Mastectomy, on the other hand, is associated with less than a 3% lifetime risk of recurrence. Therefore, treatment must be individualized for each patient.

LCIS is associated with a 1% per year bilateral risk for the development of breast cancer. Traditional management consists of close screening and follow-up. If the patient is young with a multigeneration family history of premenopausal breast cancer, a mastectomy may be warranted.

Atypical ductal hyperplasia is associated with an increased risk of subsequent cancer development. Management of this preinvasive lesion should be individualized to each patient. In patients with a positive family history and atypical ductal hyperplasia, prophylactic chemotherapy or an experimental chemoprevention trial may be warranted.

ADJUVANT THERAPY[1,8,27–30]

In the 1950s it was recognized that micrometastases existed at the time of diagnosis of breast cancer. This concept dictated the need for combined modality therapy, including both regional and systemic treatment. The role of adjuvant therapy is still being established, and its effect on mortality rate is still being defined. Adjuvant therapy consists of hormonal therapy, chemotherapy and immunotherapy. The EBCTCG meta-analysis showed in 1985 that adjuvant chemotherapy or adjuvant hormonal therapy produced significant reductions in the annual odds of recurrence and annual odds of death compared with no adjuvant systemic therapy.

Hormonal therapy

Hormonal therapy consists of the administration of tamoxifen, megestrol acetate (Megace) or other drug agents, or surgical ovarian ablation. In general hormonal manipulation on hormonally sensitive tumors is effective, with a one-fifth reduction in death rate. The NSABP Protocol B-14 concluded that there is a significant prolongation of disease-free survival in patients receiving tamoxifen treatment when compared to patients who did not receive tamoxifen. In addition, it has been found that the beneficial effects of tamoxifen therapy are most evident in patients over 50 and in women with ER-positive (estrogen receptor) tumors. Tamoxifen therapy should be begun immediately, although there is evidence that there will still be some therapeutic benefit if therapy is started more than two years after the diagnosis of breast cancer. Indirect evidence from the combined analysis of tamoxifen treatment trials has demonstrated that the benefit from two to five years of tamoxifen treatment is greater than that from duration of less than two years. In addition to reducing the risk of developing a second primary cancer, tamoxifen also has some other benefits. It acts as an agonist-antagonist to estrogen, and therefore it preserves bone mineral density and favorably alters the blood lipid profile.

Ovarian ablation has also been found to confer a significant benefit, with a 26% decreased overall risk in odds of recurrence and a decrease in mortality of 25% in premenopausal women. The effects of ovarian ablation appear to be greater when it is the only adjuvant therapy given than when it is combined with cytotoxic chemotherapy.

Chemotherapy

Cytotoxic chemotherapy trials show a reduction in death rate of approximately 30% to 35%. The efficacy of chemotherapy has been found to be greater in women younger than 50. The most beneficial regimen of chemotherapy is still being investigated; however, it has been found that polychemotherapy is superior to single-agent chemotherapy. Doxorubicin and epirubicin are currently considered to be very effective agents in metastatic breast cancer, and trials are currently ongoing to investigate the use of anthracycline-containing chemotherapy regimens. Hortobagyi and colleagues recommend six cycles of adjuvant chemotherapy with either cyclophosphamide, methotrexate and 5-fluorouracil; or 5-fluorouracil, doxorubicin and cyclophosphamide (FAC); or 5-fluorouracil, epirubicin and cyclophosphamide (FEC) as appropriate standards in patients not enrolled in clinical trials. Chemotherapy should be administered for at least six months, and trials have suggested that longer therapy does not offer any survival advantage.

The administration of high-dose chemotherapy with subsequent autologous bone marrow transplant is still being investigated, and trials are taking longer than expected because people are receiving this treatment outside of study protocols. Therefore, in patients with advanced breast cancer, this treatment regimen may prove to be beneficial, and trials are currently ongoing.

The time course in which chemotherapy should be initiated is still under investigation. The Ludwig Breast Cancer Study Group has suggested that there is no additional benefit from the initiation of adjuvant chemotherapy immediately after the surgical procedure or with a delay of three to four weeks. In addition, the sequencing of chemotherapy and radiation therapy has not been determined. Retrospective analyses have suggested that delaying radiation therapy may result in increased local recurrence, whereas other studies have suggested that early institution of adjuvant chemotherapy is imperative. Further studies are warranted.

Chemotherapy and hormonal therapy

The addition of chemotherapy to tamoxifen therapy is controversial. In most trials no disease-free or overall survival advantage was observed compared with tamoxifen alone. In the Ludwig III trial, women aged 50 and over demonstrated that the combination of chemotherapy and hormone therapy was superior to hormone therapy alone or to no adjuvant therapy. However, when the patients were stratified by ER status, the results with hormone therapy alone were equivalent to those with the combination therapy in patients with ER-positive tumors, while the combination was superior in patients with ER-negative tumors. Therefore, until further studies are completed, recommendations should be to give tamoxifen alone to low-risk, receptor-positive, postmenopausal patients and a combination of both tamoxifen and chemotherapy to those postmenopausal patients with high-risk disease.

In unselected populations of patients, the combination of oopherectomy and chemotherapy for premenopausal women appears to have no benefit over either treatment alone. The Scottish Cancer Trials Breast compared CMF (cytoxin, methotrexate and 5 fluorouracil) alone with ovarian ablation alone in premenopausal women with primary breast cancer. They found that the overall relapse-free and overall survival rates for the two groups were identical. However, when broken down by receptor status, oopherectomy was superior to chemotherapy for ER-positive tumors, and chemotherapy was superior for ER-negative patients. These results need to be confirmed in future trials.

The combination of chemotherapy and hormone therapy in premenopausal women is complicated by the overlapping effects of the regimens. For instance, about two-thirds of premenopausal women become amenorrheic during adjuvant chemotherapy. Whether amenorrhea occurs depends on age, type of cytotoxic agents used and duration of treatment. While most women younger than 30 years continue to menstruate during and after chemotherapy, more than 90% of women older than 40 years become permanently amenorrheic after cytotoxic chemotherapy. Therefore, one questions whether adding ovarian ablation to the treatment of a patient who is already amenorrheic as a consequence of adjuvant chemotherapy would result in additional benefit.

Immunotherapy

Several immunomodulators have been tried in the treatment of breast cancer. These immunomodulators include bacillus Calmette–Guerin (BCG); the methanol extracted residue of BCG (MER); levamisole; Corynebacterium parvum; interferon alfa; and polyadenylic-polyuridylic acid (poly A:U). All immunotherapy trials have failed except poly A:U. In a single study, when poly A:U was administered postoperatively as the only systemic adjuvant therapy, there was an improvement in relapse-free and overall survival rates compared with surgery alone. There are no confirmatory trials yet for poly A:U adjuvant therapy.

TOXICITY OF ADJUVANT THERAPY

Hormonal therapy

The short-term side effects of hormonal therapy with tamoxifen include hot flushes, nausea, vomiting, fluid retention, weight gain and thrombocytopenia. There has been reported a rare incidence of DVT and arterial thromboses. In addition, some patients suffer from depressive episodes (less than 5%). Finally, of substantial concern is the increased risk of endometrial cancer reported in patients using tamoxifen. Therefore, any patient on tamoxifen must have routine gynecologic examinations.

The side effects of ovarian ablation include premature menopause, the early onset of osteoporosis and adverse changes in serum lipid profile that may increase the frequency and severity of adverse cardiovascular events.

Chemotherapy

The acute side effects from chemotherapy include nausea, vomiting, anorexia, alopecia, mucositis, leukopenia, neutropenia, thrombocytopenia and an increased risk of infections. The use of alkylating agents may make premenopausal patients amenorrheic and is related to the age at time of exposure and the total dose of chemotherapy given. There does not appear to be an increased risk of secondary solid tumors after adjuvant chemotherapy, but there is an increased frequency of myelodysplastic syndromes and leukemias.

WHO SHOULD RECEIVE ADJUVANT THERAPY?

It is generally accepted that all patients with node-positive primary breast cancer should receive adjuvant therapy, usually in the form of systemic chemotherapy. In addition, node negative patients with adverse prognostic indicators that place them in the moderate- to high-risk category of distant micrometastases should receive adjuvant systemic therapy. These high-risk tumor characteristics include aneuploidy, estrogen receptor-negative, high S fraction, high HER 2, and high cathepsin D.

It is essential to remember that the benefits of adjuvant therapy must be weighed against the adverse affects of the regimen. At the University of Texas, MD Anderson Center, patients who elect not to participate in clinical trials or who are ineligible for clinical trials are managed as follows:

1. With noninvasive or microinvasive disease of any histological subtype, or invasive ductal or lobular carcinomas less than 1 cm, patients are treated with local/regional therapy, and no adjuvant systemic therapy is offered as the potential risks probably outweigh the benefits.
2. All patients younger than 50 who would benefit from adjuvant therapy are given a trial of chemotherapy.
3. Patients older than 50 with ER-positive tumors in a low-risk category are treated with tamoxifen alone.
4. Patients at high risk of recurrence are treated with combined tamoxifen and chemotherapy.
5. Patients with ER-negative tumors are treated with chemotherapy alone.
6. Patients with stage III breast cancer and patients with more than 10 positive nodes represent very high-risk groups and should be encouraged to enrol in a clinical trial for high-dose chemotherapy and autologous bone marrow transplant.

CONCLUSION

In conclusion, perimenopausal breast disease encompasses a broad spectrum of breast lesions ranging from benign to malignant disease. Breast cancer warrants particular consideration as it is the leading cause of cancer in women, which has a high mortality rate. Efforts at improving screening and diagnostic ability are currently ongoing. In addition, clinical trials are in progress investigating optimal treatment regimens for patients afflicted with breast cancer.

REFERENCES

1 Iglehart JD: The breast. In: Sabiston DC and Lyerly HK, *Textbook of Surgery. The Biological Basis of Modern Surgical Practice.* Fifteenth edition. Philadelphia: W.B. Saunders Company, 1997, pp. 555–594.
2 Bland KI, Copeland EM III: Breast. In: Schwartz SI, Shires GT, Spencer FC and Husser WC, *Principles of Surgery.* Sixth edition. New York: McGraw-Hill, 1994, pp. 531–595.
3 Wheater PR, Burkitt HG, Daniels VG: *Functional Histology. A Text and Colour Atlas.* Second edition. New York: Churchill Livingstone, 1987, pp. 304–307.

4 NCI: Fact Sheet: Benign Breast Lumps and Other Benign Breast Changes. *Oncolink* 7/95 http:// oncolink.upenn.edu/disease/breast/cancernet 1994–1997.

5 Dupont WD, Parl FF, Hartmann WH, Brinton LA *et al.*: Breast cancer risk associated with proliferative breast disease and atypical hyperplasia. *Cancer* 71: 1258–1265, 1993.

6 London SJ, Connolly JL, Schnitt SJ, Colditz GA: A prospective study of benign breast disease and the risk of breast cancer. *JAMA* 267: 941–944, 1992.

7 Meguid MM, Oler A, Numann P, Khan S: Pathogenesis-based treatment of recurring subareolar breast abscesses. *Surgery* 118: 775–782, 1995.

8 Zeiger MA, Walt AJ, Dooley WC, Wood WC: The breast. In: JC Cameron, *Current Surgical Therapy*. Fifth edition. St. Louis: Mosby-Year Book, Inc, 1995, pp. 534–569.

9 Bilimoria MM, Morrow M: The woman at increased risk for breast cancer: Evaluation and management strategies. *CA Cancer J Clin* 45: 263–278, 1995.

10 National Cancer Institute: *Oncolink* NCI fact sheet: Known factors may account for more than 40 percent of US breast cancer cases. http://oncolink.upenn.edu/disease/breast/cancernet 1994–1997.

11 Scott-Conner CEH, Schorr SJ: The diagnosis and management of breast problems during pregnancy and lactation. *Am J Surgery* 170: 401–405, 1995.

12 National Cancer Institute: *Oncolink* NCI fact sheet: Oral contraceptives and breast cancer. http:// oncolink.upenn.edu/disease/breast/cancernet 1994–1997.

13 Brinton LA, Daling JR, Liff JM *et al.*: Oral contraceptives and breast cancer risk among younger women. *JNCI* 87: 827–835, 1995.

14 Colditz GA, Hankinson SE, Hunter DJ, *et al.*: The use of estrogens and progestins and the risk of breast cancer in postmenopausal women. *N Engl J Med* 332: 1589–1593, 1995.

15 McNamee D: A change in lifestyle may prevent cancer. *Lancet* 348: 1436, 1996.

16 Bernstein L, Henderson BE, Hanisch R, Sullivan-Halley J, Ross RK: Physical exercise and reduced risk of breast cancer in young women. *JNCI* 86: 1403–1408, 1994.

17 van den Brandt PA, Goldbohm A, van't Veer P: Alcohol and breast cancer: results from the Netherlands cohort study. *Am J Epidemiol* 141: 907–915, 1995.

18 Kopans DB: The accuracy of mammographic interpretation. *N Engl J Med* 331: 1521–1522, 1994.

19 Davies RJ, A'Hern RPA, Parsons CA, Moskovic EC: Mammographic accuracy and patient age: A study of 297 patients undergoing breast biopsy. *Clin Radiol* 47: 23–25, 1993.

20 Elmore JG, Wells CK, Lee CH, Howard DH, Feinstein AR: Variability in radiologists' interpretations of mammograms. *N Engl J Med* 331: 1483–1489, 1994.

21 National Cancer Institute: *Oncolink* NCI/PDQ Physician Statement: Screening for breast cancer. http://oncolink.upenn.edu/disease/breast/cancernet 1997.

22 Janes R, Bouton MS: Initial 300 consecutive stereotactic core-needle breast biopsies by a surgical group. *Am J Surgery* 168(6): 533–537, 1994.

23 Albertini JJ, Lyman GH, Cox C, Yeatman T, Balducci L, Ku N, Shivers S, Berman C, *et al.*: Lymphatic mapping and sentinel node biopsy in the patient with breast cancer. *JAMA* 276(22): 1818–1822, 1996.

24 Moore MP, Kinne DW: The surgical management of primary invasive breast cancer. *CA Cancer J Clin* 45: 279–288, 1995.

25 Kunkler I: Scottish randomised controlled trial of conservative therapy for breast cancer. *Lancet* 348: 1458–1459, 1996.

26 Hetelekidis S, Schnitt ST, Morrow M, Harris JR: Management of ductal carcinoma in situ. *CA Cancer J Clin* 45: 244–253, 1995.

27 NCI CancerLit News: *Clinical Announcement: Adjuvant Therapy of Breast Cancer – Tamoxifen update*. National Cancer Institute. http://oncolink.upenn.edu/disease/breast/cancernet m 1994–1997.

28 Early Breast Cancer Trialists' Collaborative Group: Ovarian ablation in early breast cancer: Overview of the randomised trials. *Lancet* 348: 1189–1196, 1996.

29 Hortobagyi GN, Buzdar AU: Current status of adjuvant systemic therapy for primary breast cancer: Progress and controversy. *CA Cancer J Clin* 45: 199–226, 1995.

30 Bonadonna G, Valagussa P, Zucali R, Salvadori B: Primary chemotherapy in surgically resectable breast cancer. *CA Cancer J Clin* 45: 227–243, 1995.

8

Urinary tract infection

ZAHI N MAKHULI

INTRODUCTION

Urinary tract infections in the perimenopause period are similar to other urinary tract infections in all women, except for the slightly increased incidence which is primarily a result of the decreased estrogen level in the former. Therefore, a discussion of urinary tract infection in general will cover the subject.

Coliforms are the usual cause of these infections, being the normal flora of the bowel, but causing colonization, invasion, and damage to the urinary tract. Several reasons have been found to explain this process, including the adhesive characteristics of the bacteria and the receptive properties of the urothelial cells, modification of the vaginal fluid and the role of the normal genital flora, mainly the lactobacilli, in protecting against colonization.

ADHESIVE PROPERTIES OF THE BACTERIA AND RECEPTIVE PROPERTIES OF UROTHELIAL CELLS

The uropathogens, for example E. coli, initially colonize the vaginal mucosa[1] and move to the urethra before ascending to the bladder.[2] Adherence of the bacteria to the epithelial vaginal cell is a result of filamentous appendages called pili.[3] These pili can be variable functionally and antigenically. Two such pili have been described for E. coli: type 1 and type P, which are predominantly present in cystitis and pyelonephritis respectively. Expression of the type 1 pili in the experimental animal has been shown to be variable where the piliated bacteria will be present on the urothelial cell; however, the nonpiliated ones will be recovered in the urine. This may explain how some patients with symptoms of cystitis may have a negative urine culture.[4]

Schaeffer[5] has suggested that the surface of the urothelial cell is genetically determined and may explain recurrent urinary tract infections in some women.

MODIFICATION OF THE VAGINAL FLUID

Hormonal fluctuations have been shown to change the vaginal environment; for example, estrogen replacement therapy lowers the vaginal pH, which in turn reduces colonization[6] and subsequent urinary tract infection. Reid and associates[7] have also shown that uroepithelial cells from postmenopausal women have much more susceptibility to attract uropathogens than those from premenopausal women.

Mucus production is another factor which may be affected by hormonal changes. The quantities of mucus may either increase or decrease the adherence of uropathogens, as has been shown by Duncan and colleagues.[8]

ROLE OF GENITAL FLORA

'Bacterial interference' has been shown to act as a defense mechanism against pathogens. The intestinal tract *Clostridium difficile* will cause severe diarrhea after antibiotic-induced changes in the normal flora.[9] Similarly, any interference with normal vaginal flora has been shown to increase the possible colonization of the vaginal cells, with subsequent ascending infection per urethra to cause cystitis. Experimentally, Winberg and colleagues[10] have shown that lactobacilli alone cannot eliminate *E. coli* colonization, but the use of fresh vaginal fluid from healthy animals did. Studies on the use of lactobacilli in patients with recurrent urinary tract infections has been reported by Bruce.[11]

CLASSIFICATION AND MANAGEMENT OF URINARY TRACT INFECTIONS

It is very important to classify urinary tract infections according to their severity and site of infection in order to treat them properly. In perimenopausal and postmenopausal women, the status of their hormone levels seems to play a big role and, therefore, estrogen replacement with close clinical monitoring is essential.

Accordingly, urinary tract infections can be classified into lower (cystitis-urethritis) or upper (pyelonephritis). By far, cystitis is much more common and usually easier to treat, although it may become recurrent, with many work days lost at a significant cost. Most cystitis is caused by *E. coli* and minimal workup is required, consisting of urinalysis showing microscopic pyuria and positive leukocyte esterase dipstick. A urine culture is not necessary unless it is a recurrent infection. A three-day course of trimethoprim–sulfamethoxazole 160–800 mg respectively every twelve hours should be sufficient. In recurrent infections, a urine culture is necessary and, in addition to estrogen replacement, low-dose, long-term treatment with either nitrofurantoin 50 mg, trimethoprim 100 mg, or trimethoprim-sulfamethoxazole 40–200 mg respectively daily. Persistent unresponsive cystitis should be investigated further to rule out any anatomical problems, such as cystoceles or urethral diverticuli, and to correct these if present.

Upper urinary tract infection is a result of an ascending propagation of cystitis and presents with chills, fever and flank pain. An uncomplicated situation, that is, where no anatomical abnormalities are suspected, can be treated by oral fluoroquinolones, for example, ciprofloxacin 500 mg every 12 hours. However, if the patient is vomiting and cannot take oral medications, parenteral treatment with gentamicin (1 mg per kg every eight hours), with or without ampicillin (1 g every six hours), is initiated and changed to oral ciprofloxacin, 500 mg every 12 hours when oral intake is possible; continue for a total of 14 days.

In patients with complicated pyelonephritis, such as where calculi or obstruction is suspected, radiological investigation with an intravenous pyelogram is necessary. Any abnormalities should be corrected in order to treat the infection adequately.

In summary, the pathogenesis of urinary tract infection has been presented, emphasizing the hormonal changes in perimenopausal women. Classification and management was discussed.

REFERENCES

1 Neu HC: Urinary tract infection *Am J Med* 92: 4A,635–705,1992.
2 Stamey TA, Sexton GG: The role of vaginal colonization with enterobacterincase in recurrent urinary infections. *J Urol* 113–214,1975.
3 Klemm P: Fimbrial adhesions of *Escherichia coli. Rev Infect Dis* 7: 321,1985.
4 Schaeffer AJ. Update on the pathogenesis and management of urinary tract infection in women. *Monographs in Uro* 17: 68,1996.
5 Schaeffer AJ, Jones JM, Dunn JK: Association of *in vitro Escherichia coli* adherence to vaginal and buccal epithelial cells with susceptibility to women to recurrent urinary tract infections. *N Engl J Med* 304: 1062–1066,1981.
6 Raz R, Stamm WE: A controlled trial on intravaginal estriol in postmenopausal women with recurrent urinary tract infection. *N Engl J Med* 329–753,1981.
7 Reid G, Zorzitto ML, Bruce AW, et al.: Pathogenesis of urinary tract infection in the elderly: The role of bacterial adherence to uroepithelial cells. *Curr Microbiol* 11: 67,1984.
8 Duncan JL: Differential effects of Tamm–Horstall protein on adherence of *Escherichia coli* to transitional epithelial cells. *J Infect Dis* 158: 1379,1988.
9 Aransson B, Molby R, Nord CE: Antibacterial agents and *Clostridium difficile* in acute enteric disease: Epidimiologic data from Sweden 1980–82. *J Infect Dis* 151: 476–481,1985.
10 Weinberg J, Herthelius–Elman M, Molby R, Nord C: Pathogenesis of urinary tract infection – Experimental studies of vaginal resistence to colonization. *Pediatr Nephrol* 7: 509–514,1993.
11 Bruce AW, Reid G: Intravaginal installation of lactobacilli for prevention of recurrent urinary tract infections. *Con J Microbiol* 34: 339–343,1988.

9

Urinary stress incontinence in the perimenopause

GIOVANNI ELIA

INTRODUCTION

The prevalence of urinary incontinence is difficult to assess because of cultural and social reasons. It has been estimated that 13 million Americans are incontinent, 11 million of whom are women. Twenty-five percent of women between 30 and 59 years of age have experienced urinary incontinence;[1] 15% to 30% of individuals aged 60 or older are affected by urinary incontinence. The cost of this problem is even more staggering: $16.4 billion is spent every year in the U.S. on incontinence-related care and $1.1 billion is spent on disposable absorbent products for adults.[1] The definition of urinary incontinence as given by the International Continence Society (ICS) is the 'involuntary loss of urine which is objectively demonstrable and a social and hygienic problem.'[2] Therefore the indication for diagnostic workup and treatment plan is reserved to women whose condition is subjectively bothersome. For example, a very active young woman may be severely distressed by minimal loss of urine during physical exercise, whereas an older multipara may think that wearing pads is a normal sign of aging.

TYPES OF URINARY INCONTINENCE

Urinary incontinence may be divided in two groups: the first is related to abnormalities of the storage phase, the second to abnormalities of the voiding phase (Figure 9.1).

Stress urinary incontinence (SUI) occurs during sudden increase of intra-abdominal pressure without concomitant bladder contraction. Bladder overactivity or detrusor instability (DI) is characterized by uninhibited bladder contractions during bladder filling.

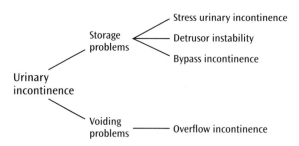

Figure 9.1 *Classification of urinary incontinence.*

Table 9.1 *Prevalence of urinary incontinence in a continence outpatient facility*

Genuine stress incontinence only	50–75%
Detrusor instability only	10–30%
Mixed genuine stress incontinence and detrusor instability	5–15%
Hyperreflexic (neurogenic bladder)	<5%
Urinary fistula or diverticulum	<5%
Retention with overflow, other voiding disorders	<5%
No incontinence demonstrated	1–10%

AUGS Quarterly Report, Vol. 7, no. 1, 1989

Mixed incontinence is a combination of the previous two. Bypass incontinence is related to anatomical abnormalities that bypass the urethral sphincteric mechanism (for example, vesico–vaginal fistula, urethral diverticulum, or ectopic ureter). Overflow incontinence is more common in men as a result of bladder outflow obstruction from benign prostatic hyperplasia. The respective prevalence of these conditions in a selected population of women attending an incontinence outpatient facility is shown in Table 9.1.

ESTROGEN AND THE LOWER URINARY TRACT

The presence of receptors for estrogen in the female lower urinary tract has been postulated for years based on the subjective improvement noted in postmenopausal women with urinary symptoms after estrogen replacement.[3–5] The urethra and vagina have in fact a common embryologic origin: the urogenital sinus. Holderegger and Keefer[6] observed the serial increase of estrogen receptor in pelvic organs (including the bladder and urethra) during early gestational stages in mice. Iosif[7] and colleagues demonstrated the existence of high-affinity estradiol receptors in the female urethra. These receptors were of the same type as those found in the vagina. The concentration of receptors in the bladder, however, was considerably lower than in the urethra. Other authors confirmed these findings[8–10] and also proved the existence of progesterone receptors in the urethra and in the bladder.[9]

The presence of a significantly high concentration of estrogen receptors in the lower urinary tract and particularly in the urethra explains the responsiveness of this organ to estrogen stimulation.

Batra and Iosif[11] and Shapiro[12] demonstrated a significant increase in the wet weight of the uterus, vagina and urethra in ovariectomized rabbits following estradiol replacement. Batra and colleagues,[13,14] in subsequent studies, observed a significant increase of blood flow in the uterus, vagina and urethra two hours after intra-arterial injection of estradiol. This effect was decreased by the simultaneous injection of progesterone.[14] At the level of the urethral epithelial lining, estrogens increase the proliferation of superficial squamous epithelium[15] exerting a general trophic action.[16,17] Estrogen replacement seems also to induce fibrosis of the connective tissue and engorgement of blood vessels surrounding the urethra.[18,19] Several studies on animal models *in vitro* and *in vivo* investigated the effect of estrogens on the spontaneous activity of the urethral smooth muscles and on the responsiveness of the adrenergic receptors.[20,21] Estrogen enhanced the sensitivity of the urethral smooth muscle through an increase in number of postjunctional alpha-2 adrenoceptors, which causes contraction of the periurethral smooth muscles.[22]

ESTROGEN REPLACEMENT

In the postmenopausal woman, the urethra is one of the organs most affected by the decrease in circulating estrogens.[16,23] Estrogen replacement therapy is administered mainly as oral pills, vaginal creams, and transdermal patch. For oral administration, natural (micronized estradiol, piperazine estrone sulfate), equine (conjugated estrogens) and synthetic estrogens (ethinylestradiol, diethylestilbestrol) are available in the U.S.[24,25]

Serum levels of estrogens (estradiol and estrone) are similar for oral administration of 0.625 mg of estrogens, conjugated estrogens or estrone and for 1 mg of micronized estradiol.[26] The intravaginal route was studied by Schiff and colleagues[27] and by Whitehead and colleagues[28] who demonstrated that serum estrone levels with intravaginal administration were three times higher than with the oral route. Heimer[29] noted in 1987 that the administration of 1 mg of estriol intravaginally or 10 mg orally would produce similar plasma levels. More recently, the transdermal administration of estradiol has been extensively studied, and it seems to produce plasma levels strictly related to the dose contained in the patch.[30,31]

The advantage of parenteral routes compared with oral is that they avoid the enterohepatic first pass, which reduces the bioavailability by up to 30%.[24] Less liver stimulation has also been noted with parenteral administration.[26] Systemic biologic effects are similar if equivalent blood levels are reached.[24] However, tissue levels in the urinary tract are higher with the vaginal application of estrogens.

ESTROGEN AND URINARY PHYSIOLOGY

The mechanism of continence in the female urethra is based on four anatomical entities: the epithelium, the connective tissue, the periurethral vascular structure, and the sphincteric mechanism of the striated and smooth muscles of the periurethra and pelvic floor.[32,15,33–38] These four factors contribute in varying degrees[38] to the urethral closure pressure and are all estrogen-sensitive.

In 1980 Rud[39] evaluated the urodynamic function of 169 continent women (aged six to 71). He noted that the maximum urethral pressure and the urethral length increased from infancy to between 20 and 25 years of age. These parameters subsequently decreased with increasing age. No changes related to varied hormone levels were noted during the menstrual cycle. Additional studies confirmed Rud's observations.[40,41] Van Geelen and coworkers[42] suggested a direct causal relationship between changes of urethral length and estradiol levels only during normal menstrual cycles. Karram and colleagues[43] did not find significant differences in urethral pressure, functional length, or cystometric parameters in women with premature ovarian failure before and after estrogen replacement therapy. However, they did find a significant increase in urethral pressure transmission to the urethra once estrogen replacement was reinstituted.

Langer and colleagues[44] demonstrated no urodynamic changes in asymptomatic women before and after six months of hypoestrogenism induced with GnRH agonist.

These studies suggest that the development of urinary incontinence in women not only is affected by estrogen deficiency but is also the consequence of more complex interactions related to the aging of anatomical structures.

DIAGNOSTIC EVALUATION

Step I: History and physical examination

Women with complaints of urinary incontinence usually present several years after the onset of their symptoms. The complaints are related to lifestyle, socioeconomic status, work schedule or leisure activity. There is no recipe for the treatment of urinary incontinence: every woman needs an individualized plan. And this plan has its main foundation on an accurate, meticulous history. Problem-focused, but also medical history, surgical, social and family history. By definition, stress incontinence occurs with sudden increase of intra-abdominal pressure; therefore the symptom will be loss of urine on coughing, sneezing, walking, lifting, exercising and so on. Often women have symptoms consistent with stress incontinence alone or associated with urgency or urge incontinence. These last symptoms are characterized by the sudden, strong need to void (urgency) that may be associated with loss of urine (urge incontinence). It is important to elicit a history of urgency, because it has been proved that in these cases cystoscopy with urodynamic testing may be necessary. Even with straightforward complaints of stress incontinence, the positive predictive value of history alone is 80%.[45] This figure may appear satisfactory from the statistical point of view but is not acceptable in the clinical setting. If the indication for surgery were based on history alone, 20% of major surgery would be performed for the wrong reason.

The medical history may disclose information such as the use of diuretics and alpha or beta blockers for essential hypertension; a history of chronic obstructive pulmonary disease, neuropathy or diabetes mellitus is also of great importance. The surgical history may help in evaluating recurrences after incontinence surgery or urinary symptoms after radical surgery or radiotherapy. Often underestimated is the social history. Knowing the time and amount of caffeine or alcohol intake, for example, may be essential in the treatment of urinary incontinence and other urinary problems. Sexual history is also important for several reasons; urinary incontinence during intercourse may be very distressing, and in some cases women abstain from sexual activity because of the embarassment. This particular problem may be caused by stress incontinence or by detrusor instability triggered during orgasm. Furthermore, the desire of the patient about preserving her sexual function is an important guide in planning pelvic reconstructive surgery.

An invaluable tool to obtain a more objective picture of the patient's voiding and drinking habits as well as of the frequency of incontinence episodes is the voiding diary or urology. This should be completed over one week; however, many women find it difficult to do it over such a long time period. Therefore two or three days may be a good compromise. The voiding diary allows the calculation of total fluid intake, amount and type of beverages (coffee, soda, juice, and so on), volume voided, number and circumstances of incontinence episodes.

After a detailed history, a urine dipstick will be necessary to screen for infection or other bladder or renal pathology. Bladder catheterization should then be performed no more than five minutes after voiding to measure the postvoid residual and thus rule out voiding dysfunction. No definite cutoff has been established to define what is a 'normal' postvoid residual. Some give absolute numbers, such as 50, 70 or 100 cc. It is better to refer the residual to the amount voided. A general rule to define a normal postvoid residual is that it should be less than 25% to 30% of the total urine obtained (amount voided plus residual). An absolute number may have a different meaning if, for example, a residual of 50 cc is obtained after a voided volume of 25 cc or 400 cc.

To rule out a subclinical neuropathy, a neurologic exam targeted to the assessment of the S2–S4 levels of the spinal cord should be performed. This is easily achieved by a test for pinprick, pressure and vibration sensation in the areas innervated by the S2–S4 dermatomes (Figure 9.2) and by the assessment of the anal and clitoral reflexes (Figure 9.3).

A physical exam should then be aimed at the assessment of genital organ estrogenization and degree of pelvic relaxation, if any. Careful evaluation of anterior and posterior vaginal walls, and uterus in the supine and standing position will unveil any pelvic organ descensus. A rectovaginal exam will allow evaluation of the anal spincter, rectovaginal septum, posterior cul-de-sac, uterosacral and cardinal ligaments. During the performance of the pelvic exam, care should be taken with the assessment of the strength of the levator ani and the ability of the patient to perform a pelvic floor muscle contraction without using accessory muscles and without performing a Valsalva maneuver. This information can be very helpful in deciding if a subject is a candidate for pelvic floor muscle exercises.

In women complaining of stress incontinence, the loss of urine can be objectively demonstrated by doing the cough stress test. The patient is asked to cough while in standing

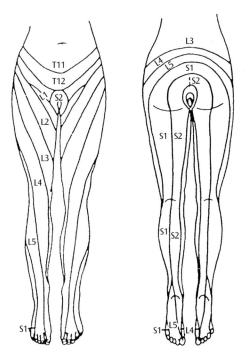

Figure 9.2 *Lower extremity sensory dermatomes.*

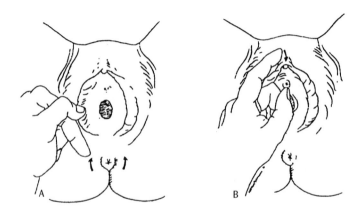

Figure 9.3 *The anal and clitoral reflexes. Gentle stroking lateral to the anus causes anal sphincter contraction (A). Gentle tapping or pressure on the clitoris causes pelvic floor contraction (B).*

position with full bladder. The diagnosis will be made by observing loss of urine from the urethra exactly at the time of the cough.

To complete the assessment of pelvic organs, a simple but invaluable test is the Q-tip test. This is performed with the patient on the examining table in lithotomy position. A well-lubricated Q-tip is advanced in the bladder and then gently withdrawn until the subtle resistance offered by the bladder neck to the cotton end is appreciated. The angle of the Q-tip with the horizontal line is measured and this is the resting angle. Then the patient is asked to perform a strong Valsalva manuever, and the new angle with the horizontal is measured. If the starting angle or the change of angle is 30 degrees or more, the test is positive. This means that the bladder neck is hypermobile and therefore suitable for surgical correction. The Q-tip test is not diagnostic for stress incontinence, but is very helpful in defining if a urethropexy is indicated.[47,48]

Step II: Urethrocystoscopy

The previously described evaluation will be sufficient to start a conservative plan of management as described in the next section of this chapter.

If the patient complains of 'irritative symptoms' such as urgency, frequency or dysuria in the absence of urinary infection, a urethrocystoscopy may be warranted. A stronger indication for urethrocystoscopy is the association of the above complaints with microscopic hematuria, a history of smoking or previous radiation therapy for genital cancer. The test in these cases will rule out bladder or urethral pathology such as polyps, diverticula, urethritis, interstitial cystitis and so on. The procedure can be performed in the office using a rigid or a flexible cystoscope. The bladder is distended with carbon dioxide or, preferably, with sterile water. Local anesthesia is usually sufficient for patient comfort.

Further evaluation with urodynamic tests will be warranted in the following circumstances: 1) failure of conservative management; 2) severe pelvic relaxation with urogenital prolapse at the level of the vaginal introitus or lower; 3) previous anti-incontinence surgery; 4) history of radiation therapy; 5) history or physical findings or neurologic dysfunction; 6) when surgical correction is planned.

Urodynamics

Urodynamics is a series of tests for the assessment of volumes and pressures in the lower urinary tract under different preplanned conditions. To assess the filling or storage phase of bladder function, the cystometry is the most important test. This is performed with the patient in the standing position while the bladder is filled with water or carbon dioxide. The pressure in the bladder is measured by a special catheter that is also used as a port for the infusion of the filling medium. During the test, the subject is asked to cough at regular intervals. The bladder pressure during the cystometry should remain at a constant value, usually around 20 cm of water. If there is an increase of bladder pressure associated with urgency, diagnosis of bladder instability (or detrusor instability) is made. Therefore the main role of the cystometry is to rule out bladder instability, which is treated with anticholinergics.

Additional information is obtained with the urethral pressure profile (Figure 9.4). This test is performed with the patient in supine position. The measuring catheter is pulled at a constant speed, so the sensor will travel from the bladder neck to the external urethral meatus. This will allow identification of the area of highest pressure in the urethra. The value obtained is called the maximum urethral pressure. The difference between the maximum urethral pressure and the bladder pressure is the maximum urethral closure pressure. This value is considered a parameter of urethral competence because it evaluates the pressure in the urethra that opposes the pressure in the bladder. If there is 20 cm or less of water, diagnosis of low urethral pressure is made. A test that complements the assessment of the storage phase is the Stress (or Valsalva) Leak Point Pressure.[46] This test is performed with the patient in standing or supine position, with 150 cc of water in the bladder or with a full bladder. Bladder and rectal pressures are measured simultaneously. The patient is asked to perform a Valsalva manuever, and the pressures measured at the time of fluid leak are recorded. A loss of urine at a pressure of 65 cm of water or less is a sign of urethral incompetence defined as intrinsic sphincteric deficiency. The urethral pressure profile and the stress leak point pressure evaluate the urethral competence using two different physiologic mechanisms. The two tests are not always consistent. The value

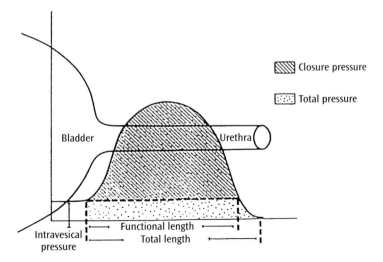

Figure 9.4 *The urethral closure pressure profile of a normal patient. The hatch lines outline the area of closure pressure, and the dotted area represents the area of total urethral pressure.*

and relationship of the two tests need further assessment. Presently they are considered complementary to the general incontinence workup.

A more sophisticated test is used to evaluate the storage phase in patients with neuropathy or after multiple surgical procedures for incontinence. This is the videocystourethrography, using either X-ray or ultrasonographic techniques. The cost and exposure to radiation limit the routine use of this technique.

The assessment of the voiding phase is performed with the uroflowmetry. This is basically the measurement of the volume of urine voided per unit of time (in ml per second). The study can be performed with instruments as simple as a stopwatch and a container or as sophisticated as a urodynamic machine with a computerized report of flow, volume and amount voided. To have a more accurate picture of the different functional features of the voiding mechanism, pressure/flow (V/Q) study should be used. This can only be performed with sophisticated equipment. The parameters measured simultaneously are bladder pressure, rectal pressure, detrusor pressure (difference between bladder pressure and abdominal pressure), flow rate and volume voided. The voiding/pressure study allows the assessment of the voiding mechanism by evaluating the intraluminal pressure generated by the detrusor muscle. In the case of incomplete bladder emptying, the diagnosis of bladder hyporeflexia versus outlet obstruction is easily made. Voiding with high intraluminal pressure is caused by outlet obstruction; low detrusor pressure during voiding, often concomitant with the increase of rectal pressure (Valsalva manuever), is consistent with bladder hyporeflexia.

Electromyography is a test that allows the diagnosis of complex voiding dysfunctions such as detrusor-sphincter dyssynergia, often found in patients with central neuropathy.

THERAPY

Nonsurgical

The treatment of women complaining of urinary incontinence can be started after the evaluation described as Step I. The history and voiding diary can give enough information to start implementing changes of medication regimen, dietary changes and changes of voiding habits. For example, diuretics for the treatment of hypertension may substantially worsen urinary incontinence that would otherwise be tolerable; alpha and beta blockers cause urethral sphincter relaxation, and it has been proved that stopping such therapies may be sufficient to treat incontinence in some women.

The same diuretic effect is exerted by coffee and caffeinated drinks as well as alcohol. Patient awareness about these effects may be all that is needed for a successful therapy.

Furthermore the above mentioned dietary and medication changes can be implemented even without a definite diagnosis. Timed voiding is the next step. This consists of voiding at a certain time interval. Timed voiding, or bladder drill, works mainly through two mechanisms: first, it keeps the bladder at low filling volume, thus minimizing the risk of involuntary urine loss; second, in patients with urgency and urge incontinence, it is a method to 'retrain' the bladder. Voluntary control over the micturition mechanism is achieved by having the patient void at a time interval that is sightly longer than her baseline (as noted in the voiding diary). The time between voiding is then increased gradually as it is tolerated by the patient, up to about three hours.

Pelvic muscle exercises are the next treatment option for urinary incontinence. These are effective in 50% to 60% of women with stress incontinence, but can be started without a definite diagnosis as long as overflow incontinence is ruled out. A postvoid residual measurement will be sufficient. Pelvic muscle exercises were first introduced by Dr. Kegel in 1948[49] and have the goal of increasing the tone and strength of contraction of the levator ani. In order to obtain the best results, the patient should be instructed while performing a pelvic exam and should be involved in a program with close follow-up and office sessions. There are many methods of performing the exercises and all of them are similarly efficacious. The one we favor consists of performing a series of five-second contractions, followed by ten-second relaxation for ten minutes, four times a day. This is an intensive program that should be followed for three months with frequent office visits. If the results are satisfactory, a maintenance regimen with exercises once or twice a day should be continued indefinitely. It is essential to make sure that the pelvic muscle contraction is performed without a concomitant Valsalva manuever and without accessory muscle involvement.[50]

The use of vaginal cones is also aimed at strengthening the levator ani.[51] The patient buys a set of cones of increasing weight but of the same size. She is instructed to start with the lightest cone and hold it in the vagina for about twenty minutes once or twice a day. As her levator ani becomes stronger she will use heavier cones. This method has the advantage of requiring less instruction and reinforcement; however, it can only be performed in a private environment.

Another technique that uses basic physiologic principles is biofeedback.[52] By definition, biofeedback is the creation of a feedback signal that makes the individual aware of physiologic changes in response to a voluntary action. The simplest biofeedback technique is to perform a pelvic exam while the subject contracts her pelvic floor muscles. A statement about the strength of the contraction is, of itself, a biofeedback. A slightly more sophisticated level is achieved with a perineometer. This instrument measures the increase of intravaginal pressure in response to a pelvic muscle contraction. The measuring probe is a small cylindrical balloon that is placed in the vagina. The biofeedback effect is achieved when the pressure gauge is placed in front of the patient, who can then observe the magnitude of her effort. More complex biofeedback units use measurement of electrical changes in pelvic muscle fibers, displayed on a high-resolution monitor. This technique can be used for the treatment of stress and urge incontinence. In the first case the goal is to strengthen the pelvic floor muscles; this is achieved by measuring pressure changes or changes in electric potentials in the vagina. For the treatment of urge incontinence with bladder instability a probe is placed in the vagina and a pressure transducer is placed in the bladder. The bladder is then filled with water, and at the onset of a bladder contraction (which can be seen on a monitor), the patient is asked to contract the pelvic floor in order to inhibit the increase of bladder pressure.

Electrical stimulation is another management option for the treatment of stress incontinence. It is usually performed by inserting in the vagina a device connected to a small unit that delivers a faradic current. Amplitude and frequency of the current can be adjusted, based on patient feeling and comfort. The results with this technique have been promising.[53]

The female urethra is under alfa-adrenergic control. The urethral smooth muscle tone increases under sympathetic stimulation. Based on this principle, alpha-adrenergic drugs can be used for the treatment of stress incontinence. The most common used are phenylpropanolamine and pseudoephedrine. Close monitoring of the blood pressure is suggested when prescribing these medications to elderly people or to individuals with essential hypertension.

ESTROGENS IN THE TREATMENT OF STRESS URINARY INCONTINENCE

Urinary incontinence in perimenopausal women, whether associated with aging of the pelvic support structures or with detrusor instability, is worsened by hypoestrogenism.

For many years the effects of estrogen replacement on urogenital symptoms have been empirically proven. With the advent of urodynamics, attempts have been made to identify and measure the changes in the urinary tract induced by estrogens. The first report comes from Salmon and colleagues[4] who, in 1941, treated 16 postmenopausal women with intramuscular injections of estrogens for four weeks. Significant improvement was noted relative to dysuria, frequency and urgency, which were the primary complaints of the patients.

Other authors subsequently reported subjective relief of urinary symptoms with estrogen replacement in postmenopausal women[54-60] (Table 9.2). Faber and Heidenreich[5] were the first to monitor urodynamic parameters to evaluate objectively the efficacy of estrogen replacement therapy in patients with stress incontinence. They found an increase of urethral pressure and subjective improvement after administration of estriol. Additional studies performed with different estrogen regimens in patients with stress incontinence showed improvements of the urodynamic parameters associated with clinical improvement[3,60-62]

Rud[3] studied prospectively the effect of estrogen and progesterone in continent and stress incontinent patients, and reported significant improvement of stress incontinence in women receiving oral estrogens. Twenty–four women with stress urinary incontinence were randomly given estradiol valerate, 4 mg daily for three weeks, or estriol, 8 mg daily for three weeks, while a control group received progesterone only. Estrogen treatment resulted in significant increase in urethral pressure, significant increase in functional length and significant improvement in abdominal pressure transmission ratio to the urethra in 18 of the 24 patients. These improved urodynamic parameters correlated highly with patients' subjective improvement. Women receiving progesterone only showed no clinical or urodynamic improvement.

Bhatia and colleagues[60] reported in a prospective study that estrogen vaginal cream (2 gm per day for six weeks) resulted in cure or significant improvement of stress incontinence in 54% of cases studied. Estrogen vaginal cream positively affected incontinent women by increasing urethral closure pressure.

Hilton and Stanton[61] studied prospectively the effect of estrogen vaginal cream (conjugated estrogen, 2 gm daily for four weeks) in women with stress incontinence. They found significant improvement in the symptoms of urinary incontinence in the group receiving estrogen vaginal cream. Improvement in urinary symptoms was associated with significant increase in urethral pressure transmission ratio to the urethra after estrogen treatment[61] (Table 9.3).

Fantl and colleagues[63] compared women already on estrogens with untreated women. Both groups had complaints of urinary incontinence, and no statistically significant urodynamic differences in urethral closure pressure and functional length were found. However, the authors reported a decrease in urine loss in women with detrusor instability receiving estrogen replacement, and a decrease of the volume of fluid lost during incontinence episodes in the estrogen-treated patients.[63] Nineteen of the 23 women in this study received estrogen in the form of Premarin PO.

In 1988, Kinn and Lindskog[64] reported increased urethral pressure in patients with initial low urethral pressure who received estrogen therapy.

Bergman and colleagues[15] studied prospectively the clinical and urodynamic effects of estrogen vaginal cream (conjugated estrogen, 2 gm per day for six weeks) in postmenopausal

Table 9.2 *Clinical changes in postmenopausal incontinent women receiving estrogen replacement therapy*

Author		No. of patients	Estrogen	Route	Improved
Salmon UJ et al.	1941	16	–	IM	Urgency frequency dysuria Incontinence
Musiani U	1972	110	Quinestradiol	Oral	Stress incontinence
Caine M and Raz S	1973	40	Conjugated equine	Oral	Stress incontinence
Schleyer-Saunders E	1976	100	Estradiol	Implants	Stress incontinence
Heidenreich J and Faber P	1977	41	Estriol	Oral	Stress incontinence
Rud T	1980	30	Estradiol or estriol	Oral	Stress incontinence
Mohr JA et al.	1983	46	Conjugated equine	Oral & vaginal	Urgency frequency Stress incontinence
Fantl AJ et al.	1988	72	Conjugated equine	Oral &/or vaginal	Sensory threshold nocturia

Table 9.3 *Effects of vaginal estrogen replacement*

Author		No. of patients	Estrogen	Clinical response
Hilton P and Stanton SL	1983	10	Conjugated equine	Improved stress incontinence
Bhatia NN et al.	1989	11	Conjugated equine	Improved stress incontinence
Foidart JM et al.	1991	109	Estriol (sustained release)	Improved dysuria Urgency frequency

Table 9.4 *Effects of estrogens on postmenopausal women: placebo-control studies*

Author		No. of patients	Estrogen	Route	Clinical response	Urodynamic parameters
Judge TG et al.	1969	20	Quinestradiol	Oral	Improved incontinence	Not available
Walter S et al.	1978	29	Estradiol	Oral	Improved urge incontinence	No change
Samsioe G et al.	1985	34	Estriol	Oral	Improved urge & mixed incontinence	Not available
Wilson PD et al.	1987	36	Piperazine estrone sulfate	Oral	No change	No change
Cardozo L et al.	1990	46	Estradiol	Implant	No change	No change*
Foidart JM et al.	1991	109	Estriol dysuria	Vaginal	Improved frequency	Not available
Fantl AJ et al.	1996	83	Conjugated equine estrogens	Oral	No change	No change

* Objective improvement of bladder base descent

Table 9.5 *Effect of estrogens combined with alpha-sympathomimetics in women with stress urinary incontinence*

Author	No. of patients	Estrogen	Route	Alpha agonist	Clinical effects
Beisland HO et al., 1984	20	Estriol	Vaginal	PPA*	8/20 cured, 9/20 improved, 1/20 unchanged
Kinn A and Lindskog M, 1988	36	Estriol	Oral	PPA	Reduced leakage episodes by 40%, 28% cured, 53% improved
Ahlstrom K et al., 1990	29	Estriol	Oral	PPA	Reduced leakage episodes by 28%, 13/29 subjective improvement
Ek A et al., 1980	13	Estradiol	Oral	Norephedrine	Markedly improved

* PPA, Phenylpropanolamine

women with stress urinary incontinence. More than 50% of women receiving estrogen vaginal cream were significantly improved or cured.

Despite so much interest in this matter, only a few randomized placebo-control studies have been found in the literature (Table 9.4). Samsioe and colleagues[65] studied 34 patients in a prospective, double-blind, crossover study. He evaluated the effects of estriol given in a single daily dose of 3 mg versus a placebo over a period of three months. The clinical results in women treated with estrogen were excellent for symptoms of urgency and mixed incontinence and less so for stress urinary incontinence. Foidart and colleagues[66] studied the effect of vaginal estrogens in alleviating urogenital complaints. A total of 109 post-menopausal women were enrolled in a placebo-control, double-blind study. Estriol (E_3) vaginal suppository versus placebo were used twice a week for a six-month study period. The estrogen therapy resulted in significant relief of the urinary symptoms of urgency and stress incontinence. These two studies[65,66] based their observations on subjective complaints with no objective urodynamic studies.

Wilson and colleagues[67] studied 36 postmenopausal patients in a prospective double-blind trial on the effect of piperazine estrone sulfate (1.5 mg tablets for one to two weeks) versus matching placebo for stress incontinence using clinical and urodynamic criteria. After six weeks of treatment there was a significant reduction in the number of pad changes per day in the estrogen-treated patients. Urodynamic parameters did not change significantly. Cardozo,[34] using clinical and urodynamic data, observed significant improvement of bladder base descent on videocystourethrography in stress incontinent women treated with estrogens, although other urodynamic parameters did not change significantly. Walter and colleagues,[68] in a double-blind clinical trial, noted improvement in urgency and urge incontinence in women receiving estrogens. Estrogen effects in women with stress urinary incontinence were not significant.

The latest study reported by Fantl and colleagues was conducted with very strict scientific criteria.[69] The subjects had urodynamic diagnosis of stress incontinence, bladder instability or both. In the study group, conjugated estrogens were used in the oral dose of 0.625 mg daily, associated for 10 days each month with 10 mg of medroxyprogesterone acetate. The subjects were randomly allocated to study or placebo group. Subjects and investigators were blinded to the allocation. The study was carried over three months. No difference was found between the two groups in subjective complaints, amount of fluid loss and urodynamic parameters.

The effect of estrogens combined with alpha-adrenergic drugs in patients with genuine stress incontinence has also been studied (Table 9.5). Investigators using phyenylpropano-lamine found that combination therapy significantly increased urethral pressure[64,70,71] and improved the leakage episodes.[70,71] Beisland and colleagues[71] reported a 40% complete cure rate after combination therapy. Ek and coworkers[72] obtained similar results with norephe-drine.

Kinn and Lindskog,[64] in a prospective study, observed 36 postmenopausal women with stress incontinence. Women were randomly treated with oral estriol, 2 mg and phenylpro-panolamine, 50 mg twice daily, alone and in combination. After an initial four-week single-blind period with phenylpropanolamine, either estriol or estriol and phenylpropanolamine were given randomly for a four-week period, in a crossover design. Both regimens resulted in a significant increase in urethral pressure and significantly reduced urinary loss by 35% (measured by objective urodynamic testing). The number of leakage episodes and leakage amount were reduced by estriol or phenylpropanolamine given separately (28%) or when given as combined therapy (40%).

Ahlstrom and colleagues[70] studied 79 postmenopausal women with stress incontinence in a prospective, randomized, double-blind, crossover study. Women received 4 mg of estriol a day in addition to either 50 mg of phenylpropanolamine twice daily or a placebo for a period of six weeks. The number of leakage episodes was reduced by 28% with combined treatment. Both combined treatment and estriol alone reduced significantly the incidence of urinary incontinence complaints.

Different routes of estrogen administration seem to have different impacts on the effectiveness of the therapy. These differences can be related not only to up to a 30% decrease in bioavailability secondary to the first pass through the enterohepatic system, but also to the more efficient metabolism of the estrone through the vaginal mucosa.[28]

There seems to be a different impact of hormone replacement therapy in patients with genuine stress urinary incontinence, as compared with patients with urge incontinence. The latter group benefits more in terms of subjective improvement of symptoms and threshold of involuntary detrusor contractions. The combination of hormone replacement and alpha-adrenergic drugs seems to be more effective than estrogen alone. The vaginal route of administration of estrogens was found to be more advantageous than the oral one in terms of dose-related effects.

PESSARIES

The use of vaginal pessaries for the treatment of stress incontinence has been an old practice used mainly in women who were not suited for surgical intervention because of age and medical problems. This practice has been neglected for several years because anesthesia techniques have dramatically decreased surgical morbidity and mortality. In recent years there has been an increased demand for conservative management of stress incontinence, mainly due to attempts to reduce costs and prolonged absence from working activity. Numerous types of pessaries specifically designed for incontinence are now available. Strong motivation and manual dexterity are required for the fitting and the safe use of these devices. The pessary should be fitted so the patient does not have vaginal discomfort, making sure she has unobstructed voiding. After fitting, a short-term follow-up is necessary two or three days later; then the patient should be seen after two or three weeks to look for erosion of the vaginal mucosa. If the woman can remove the pessary and reinsert it, she should do it every evening. If the patient cannot master insertion and removal, she has to be seen on a monthly basis for pessary removal and cleansing. The patient should always be instructed to report vaginal discharge or bleeding.

Surgical therapy

When conservative management fails to achieve satisfactory results, stress urinary incontinence is best treated with surgical intervention. There are more than 150 procedures for stress incontinence, mostly aimed at the suspension of the bladder neck and proximal urethra: urethropexy. The most common procedures can be divided in three groups, based on the anatomical approach: 1) vaginal urethral plication; 2) needle suspensions; and 3) retropubic suspensions. The first group is basically represented by the time-honored Kelly plication; this procedure has been proved in comparative studies not to be as effective as others with a vaginal or retropubic approach (Table 9.6).

There is a large number of needle suspensions which derive mainly from individual modifications of three basic procedures created by Pereyra, Raz and Stamey (Figure 9.5). These are performed with a dual approach: a vaginal dissection and placement of non-absorbable sutures in different structures (according to each procedure) at the level of the bladder neck bilaterally; this is followed by the withdrawal of the sutures through the rectus fascia in the suprapubic area using special suture carriers. The abdominal stage is accom-

Table 9.6 *Comparative studies on procedures for stress incontinence*

Author	Vaginal	Needle suspension	Retropubic	F/U
Well (1984)	57%	50%	91%	> 6 mo
Bergman (1989)	68%	69%	88%	1 yr
Stanton (1979)	36%	–	84%	> 6 mo
Van Geleen (1988)	44%	–	85%	1–2 yrs
Bhatia (1985)	–	85%	98%	1 yr
Mundy (1983)	–	40%	73%	> 6 mo
Beck (1991)	94%	–	–	> 2 yrs
Bergman (1995)	37%	43%	82%	5 yrs

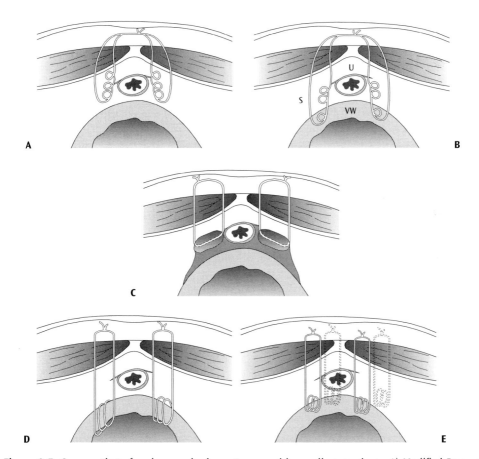

Figure 9.5 *Cross-section of various anchoring sutures used in needle procedures. A) Modified Pereyra: helical stitch through paraurethral ligament and detached endopelvic fascia. B) Raz procedure: helical stitch through detached endopelvic fascia and anchored in vaginal wall. C) Stamey procedure: buttresses are placed in the pubocervicovesical fascia on each side of the bladder neck. D) Gittes procedure: stitches through the full thickness of the vaginal wall. E) Muzsnai procedure: two stitches on either side through vaginal wall excluding epithelium.*

plished through a small suprapubic skin incision. The sutures are then tied above the rectus fascia which constitutes the suspending structure. An intraoperative cystoscopy is mandatory to rule out placement of sutures through the bladder. Success rates of these procedures are shown in Table 9.6.

The retropubic suspensions use an abdominal incision to enter the space of Retzius. Two are the most common and the ones that have gone through the test of time: the Marshall–Marchetti–Kranz (MMK), and the Burch urethropexy. The former consists of placing two sutures on each side of the endopelvic fascia in closed proximity to the bladder neck and proximal urethra. Absorbable or permanent material can be used. The sutures are then secured to the periostium in the posterior aspect of the symphysis pubis directly ventrally to the bladder neck and urethra. The most common complications and success rates are shown in Table 9.7. The MMK is often associated with the concept of osteitis pubis, but the occurrence of this complication in the gynecologic community has been overestimated. The Burch follows a similar approach, with the difference that the sutures are placed more laterally in the endopelvic fascia and then secured to the ileo-pectineal ligament (Cooper's ligament).[73] Absorbable or permanent material can be used. Success rates and complications of the Burch urethropexy are reported in Table 9.8. Recently the laparoscopic approach has been used to perform the above-described retropubic procedures. Numerous techniques have been described, some using mesh and staples, some using sutures, as in the open procedure, all substantially similar to the basic open procedures. Long-term success rates are not presently available.

The problem of SUI with intrinsic urethral sphincter deficiency requires a different surgical approach.[74] When hypermobility of the bladder neck is identified, the procedures to perform are a suburethral sling, Burch with Ball urethral plication, or the vaginal wall sling.

The suburethral sling is performed through a dual approach. First the anterior vaginal wall is dissected, then the sling is secured at the level of the bladder neck. For the sling, autologous fascia can be used, harvested from the fascia lata or from the rectus abdominis

Table 9.7 *Marshall–Marchetti–Krantz procedure*

	Patients	Follow-up	Success (%)	Complications
Marshall et al., 1949	38	1–35 months	74 (18 improved)	Wound infection 5.2% Osteitis pubis 2.6% Osteitis pubis 3.2% Urinary tract infection 10.4%
Lee et al., 1976	549	2–16 yrs	90.5	Wound infection 8.7% Voiding difficulty 2%
Riggs, 1986	411	6 mo–16 yrs	85 (9 improved)	Osteitis pubis 3%

Table 9.8 *Burch colposuspension*

	Patients	Follow-up	Success (%)	Complications
Burch, 1968	143	1–5 yrs	93	Enterocele 7.6%
Stanton, 1979	180	6 mo–2 yrs	87	Detrusor instability 2.8%
Eriksen et al., 1990	58	5 yrs	67 (cure) 21 (improved)	Detrusor instability 18% Enterocele 10%

muscle fascia[75] Artificial material such as Gore-Tex has also been used,[76] but with a substantial rate of rejection or erosion through bladder or urethra. The space of Retzius is then reached vaginally, through sharp dissection of the endopelvic fascia. A laparotomy incision is made suprapubically, and each end of the sling is pulled just underneath the rectus abdominis fascia. The sling is then secured to this fascia with permanent sutures. Care must be taken to avoid excessive tension on the sling, because it may result in permanent urinary retention or erosion through the urethra or bladder neck. To assess the degree of correction, a Q-tip is inserted in the urethra. The sling, when tied, should place the Q-tip from a positive angle with the horizontal line to a 0 degree angle. A negative angle may result in overcorrection.

The Ball urethral plication consists of placing two or three absorbable sutures in the periurethral tissues in order to taper the proximal urethra and bladder neck. Results of the Burch–Ball in women with low urethral pressure have been similar to the ones reported for the Burch in women with normal urethral pressure.[77]

The vaginal wall sling is an advancement of the needle suspensions. It is performed by dissecting the anterior vaginal wall, leaving a patch of vagina nondissected, under the bladder neck and proximal urethra.[78] Sutures are placed in each corner of the patch and pulled through the Retzius space, as is done in needle suspensions. The sutures are secured to the rectus abdominis fascia. The vaginal wall is then approximated over the vaginal patch. This procedure is more popular among urologists, and its success rate has been described in the 90% range in noncomparative studies.[78] The most common concern raised by gynecologists is related to inclusion cysts arising from the buried vaginal mucosa. The issue has been addressed in the published studies: no inclusion cyst formation was reported.

When intrinsic urethral sphincter deficiency is found in the absence of bladder neck mobility, periurethral collagen injection is the treatment of choice.[79] This procedure has been widely publicized in the lay literature as the panacea for urinary incontinence. In truth, the indication for such a procedure is present in 10% to 15% of women with stress incontinence. The material used is cross-linked bovine collagen (Gax) that is injected at the level of the bladder neck in increasing amounts until complete coaptation of the urethral mucosa is achieved. The injection can be performed through the urethral mucosa with a special delivery system attached to a cystoscope. It can also be done by advancing a 20-gauge spinal needle in the periurethral tissues up to the bladder neck; cystoscopic guidance is also necessary with this technique. Collagen injections can be performed in an office setting as well as in an ambulatory surgery center. The success rate ranges from 50% to 80% at one to two years. Several sessions may be necessary for optimal results.[79–81]

REFERENCES

1 Urinary Incontinence Guideline Panel: *Urinary Incontinence in Adults*: Clinical Practice Guideline AHCPR Pub. No. 92–0038. Rockville, MD: Agency for Health Care Policy and Research, Public Health Service, U.S. Department of Health and Human Services, March 1992.

2 Abrams P, Blaivas JG, Stanton SL, Andersen JT: Standardization of terminology: the standardization of terminology of lower urinary tract function recommended by the International Continence Society. *Int Urogynecol J* 1: 45–48,1990.

3 Rud T: The effect of estrogens and gestagens on the urethral pressure profile in urinary continent and stress incontinent women. *Acta Obstet Gynecol Scand* 59: 265,1980.

4 Salmon UJ, Walter RI, Geist SA: The use of estrogens in the treatment of dysuria and incontinence in postmenopausal women. *Am J Obstet Gynecol* 42: 845,1941.

5 Faber P, Heidenreich J: Treatment of stress incontinence with estrogen in postmenopausal women. *Urol Int* 32: 221,1977.

6 Holderegger C, and Keefer D: The ontogeny of the mouse estrogen receptor: The pelvic region. *Am J Anat* 177: 285,1986.

7 Iosif CS, Batra SC, Ek A, *et al.*: Estrogen receptors in the human female lower urinary tract. *Am J Obstet Gynecol* 141: 817,1981.

8 Walters MD, Chamness GC: Estrogen receptors in rabbit urethra and bladder. 7th Annual Meeting of the Gynecologic Urology Society. Montreal, 1996.

9 Batra SC, Josif CS: Progesterone receptors in the female lower urinary tract. *J Urol* 138: 1301,1987.

10 Schulze H, and Barrack ER: Immunocytochemical localization of estrogen receptors in the normal male and female canine urinary tract and prostate. *Endocrinology* 121: 1773,1987.

11 Batra SC, Josif CS: Female urethra: A target for estrogen action. *J Urol* 129: 418,1983.

12 Shapiro E: Effect of estrogens on the weight and musearinic cholinergic receptor density of the rabbit bladder and urethra. *J Urol* 135: 1084,1986.

13 Batra S, Bjellin L, Sjogren C, *et al.*: Increase in blood flow of the female rabbit urethra following low dose estrogens. *J Urol* 136: 1360,1986.

14 Batra S, Bjellin L, Josif S, *et al.*: Effect of oestrogen and progesterone on the blood flow in the lower urinary tract of the rabbit. *Acta Physiol Scand* 123: 191,1985.

15 Bergman A, Karram MM, and Bhatia NN: Changes in urethral cystology following estrogen administration. *Gynecol Obstet Invest* 29: 211,1990.

16 Ulmsten U, and Stormby N: Evaluation of the urethral mucosa before and after oestrogen treatment in postmenopausal women with a new sampling technique. *Gynecol Obstet Invest* 24: 208: 1987.

17 Bo von Schoultz: Estrogens and urogenital epithelial function. *Acta Obstet Gynecol Scand* 140(Suppl): 28,1987.

18 Kuroda H, Kohrogi T, Uchida N, *et al.*: Urinary retention induced by estrogen injections in mice: An analytical model. *J Urol* 134: 1268,1985.

19 Yokoyama M, Fukutani K, Kuawamura T, *et al.*: Structure of the anterior urethra following estrogen therapy in patients with prostatic cancer. *Urol Int* 38: 247,1983.

20 Callahan SM, Creed KE: The effects of estrogens on spontaneous activity and responses to phenylephrine of the mammalian urethra. *J Physiol Lond* 358: 35,1985.

21 Creed KE: Effect of hormones on urethral sensitivity to phenylephrine in normal and incontinent dogs. *Res Vet Sci* 34: 177,1983.

22 Larsson B, Andersson KE, Batra S, *et al.*: Effects of estradiol on norepinephrine-induced contraction, alfa adrenoceptor number and norepinephrine content in the female rabbit urethra. *J Pharmacol Exp Ther* 229: 557,1984.

23 Mishell DR, Jr.: Estrogen replacement therapy: An overview. *Am J Obstet Gynecol* 161(Part 2): 1825,1989.

24 Notelovitz M: Estrogen replacement therapy: Indications, contraindications, and agent selection. *Am J Obstet Bynecol* 161(Part 2): 1932,1989.

25 Stumpf PG: Pharmacokinetics of estrogen. *Obstet Gynecol* 75(Suppl): 9S,1990.

26 Lobo RA: Absorption and metabolic effects of different types of estrogens and progestogens. *Obstet Gynecol Clin North Am* 14: 143,1987.

27 Schiff I, Tulchinsky D, Ryan KJ: Vaginal absorption of estrone and 17 beta-estradiol. *Fertil Steril* 28: 1063,1977.

28 Whitehead MI, Minardi J, Kitchin Y, *et al.*: Systemic absorption of oestrogen, Premarin, vaginal cream. In: *The Role of Oestrogen/Progesterone in the Management of the Menopause*, ID Cook, ed. Lancaster, England: MJP Press.

29 Heimer GM: Estriol in the postmenopause. *Acta Obstet Gynecol Scand* Suppl.139: 4,1987.

30 Scott RT Jr., Ross B, Anderson C, *et al.*: Pharmacokinetics of percutaneous estradiol: A crossover study using a gel and transdermal system in comparison with oral micronized estradiol. *Obstet Gynecol* 77: 758,1991.

31 Holst J, Cajander S, Carlstrom K, *et al.*: Percutaneous estrogen replacement therapy: Effects of circulating estrogens, gonadotropins, and prolactin. *Acta Obstet Gynecol Scand* 62: 49,1983.

32 DeLancey JOL: Correlative study of paraurethral anatomy. *Obstet Gynecol* 69: 91,1986.

33 Versi E, Cardozo LD, Studd JWW, *et al.*: Internal urinary sphincter in maintenance of female continence. *Br Med J* 292: 166,1986.

34 Cardozo L: Role of estrogens in the treatment of female urinary incontinence. *J Am Geriatr Soc* 38: 326,1990.

35 Zinner NR, Sterling AM, Ritter RC: Role of inner urethral softness in urinary incontinence. *Urology* 16: 115,1980.

36 Asmussen M, Ulmsten U: On the physiology of continence and patho-physiology of stress incontinence in the female. In *Controversies in Gynecology and Obstetrics*, vol. 10. Basel: S Karger, AG, 1983, pp. 32–50.

37 Rud T, Andersson KE, Asmussen M, *et al.*: Factors maintaining the intraurethral pressure in women. *Invest Urol* 17: 343,1980.

38 Raz S, Caine M, Zeigler M: The vascular component in the production of intraurethral pressure. *J Urol* 108: 93,1972.

39 Rud T: Urethral pressure profile in continent women from childhood to old age. *Acta Obstet Gynecol Scand* 59: 331,1980.

40 Sorensen S, Knudsen UB, Kirkeby HJ, *et al.*: Urodynamic investigations in healthy fertile females during the menstrual cycle. *Scand J Urol Nephrol* 114(Suppl.): 28,1988.

41 Sorensen S, Waechter PB, Constantinou CE, *et al.*: Urethral pressure and pressure variations in healthy fertile and postmenopausal women with reference to the female sex hormones. *J Urol* 146: 1434,1991.

42 van Geelen JM, Doesburg WH, Thomas CM, *et al.*: Urodynamic studies in the normal menstrual cycle: The relationship between hormonal changes during the menstrual cycle and the urethral pressure profile. *Am J Obstet Gynecol* 141: 384,1981.

43 Karram MM, Yeko TR, Sauer MV, *et al.*: Urodynamic changes following hormonal replacement therapy in women with premature ovarian failure. *Obstet Gynecol* 74: 208,1989.

44 Langer R, Golan A, Neuman M, *et al.*: The absence and effect of induced menopause by gonadotropin releasing hormone analogs on lower urinary tract symptoms and urodynamic parameters. *Fertil Steril* 55: 751,1991.

45 Bergman A, Bader K: Reliability of the patient's history in the diagnosis of urinary incontinence. *Int J Gynecol Obstet* 32: 255–59,1990.

46 Wan J, McGuire EJ, Bloom DA, Ritchey ML: Stress leak point pressure: A diagnostic tool for incontinent children. *J Urol* 150: 700–702,1993.

47 Walters MD, Diaz K: Q-tip test: A study of continent and incontinent women. *Obstet Gynecol* 70: 208–211,1987.

48 Bergman A, Koonings PP, Ballard CA: Negative Q-tip test as a risk factor for failed incontinence surgery in women. *J Reprod Med* 34: 193–197,1989.

49 Kegel AH: Progressive resistance exercise in the functional restoration of the perineal muscles. *Am J Obstet Gyneccol* 56: 238–48,1948.

50 Elia G, Bergman A: Pelvic muscle exercises: When do they work? *Obstet Gynecol* 81: 283–286,1993.

51 A randomised trial of vaginal cones and pelvic floor exercises in the management of genuine stress incontinence. *Neurourol Urodynam* 10: 393–94,1991.

52 Glavind K, Walter S, Nohr S: Biofeedback training of the pelvic floor muscles in the treatment of stress urinary incontinence. *Neurourol Urodynam* 8: 435–36,1989.

53 Sand PK, Richardson DA, Staskin DR, *et al*.: Pelvic floor electrical stimulation in the treatment of genuine stress incontinence: A multicenter, placebo–controlled trial. *Am J Obstet Gynecol* 173: 72–79,1995.

54 Ouslander JG, Sier HC: Drug therapy for geriatric urinary incontinence. *Clin Ger Med* 2(4): 789,1986.

55 Battcock TM, Castleden CM: Pharmacological treatment or urinary incontinence. *Br Med Bull* 46: 147,1990.

56 Mohr JA, Rogers J Jr., Brown JN, *et al*.: Stress urinary incontinence: A simple and practical approach to diagnosis and treatment. *J Am Geriatr Soc* 31: 476,1983.

57 Jansson I: Gynecological problems in elderly women, practical aspects, treatment, care program. *Acta Obstet Gynecol Scand* Suppl.140: 60,1988.

58 Musiani U: A partially successful attempt of medical treatment of urinary stress incontinence in women. *Urol Int* 27: 405,1972.

59 Schleyer-Saunders E: Hormone implants for urinary disorders in postmenopausal women. *J Am Geriatr Soc* 24: 337,1976.

60 Bhatia NN, Bergman A, Karram MM: Effects of estrogen on urethral function in women with urinary incontinence. *Am J Obstet Gynecol* 160: 176,1989.

61 Hilton P, Stanton SL: The use of intravaginal oestrogen cream in genuine stress incontinence. *Br J Obstet Gynecol* 90: 940,1983.

62 Caine M, Raz S: *The Role of Female Hormones in Stress Incontinence*. Proceedings of the 16th Congress of the International Society of Urology, Amsterdam, 1973.

63 Fantl AJ, Wyman JF, Anderson RL, *et al*.: Postmenopausal urinary incontinence: Comparison between nonestrogen-supplemented and estrogen-supplemented women. *Obstet Gynecol* 71: 823,1988.

64 Kinn A, Lindskog M: Estrogens and phenylpropanolamine in combination for stress urinary incontinence in postmenopausal women. *Urology* 32: 273,1988.

65 Samsioe G, Jansson I, Mellstrom D, *et al*.: The occurrence, nature, and treatment of urinary incontinence in a 70 year old female population. *Maturitas* 7: 335,1985.

66 Foidart JM, Vervliet J, Buytaert PH: Efficacy of sustained-release vaginal estriol in alleviating urogenital and systemic climateric complaints. *Maturitas* 13: 99,1991.

67 Wilson PD, Faragher B, Butler B, *et al*.: Treatment with oral piperazine oestrone sulfate for genuine stress incontinence in postmenopausal women. *Br J Obstet Gynaecol* 94: 568,1987.

68 Walter S, Wolf H, Barlebo H, *et al*.: Urinary incontinence in postmenopausal women treated with oestrogens: A double-blind clinical trial. *Urol Int* 33: 135,1978.

69 Fantl aJ, Bump RC, Robinson D, *et al*.: Efficacy of estrogen supplementation in the treatment of urinary incontinence. *Obstet Gynecol* 88: 765–49, 1996.

70 Ahlstrom K, Sandah B, Sjoberg B, *et al*.: Effect of combined treatment with phenylpropanolamine and estriol, compared with estriol treatment alone, in post-menopausal women with stress urinary incontinence. *Gynecol Obstet Invest* 30: 37,1990.

71 Beisland HO, Fossberg E, Moer A, *et al*.: Urethral sphincteric insufficiency in postmenopausal females: Treatment with phenylpropanolamine and estriol separately and in combination. *Urol Int* 39: 211,1984.

72 Ek A, Andersson KE, Gullberg B, *et al*.: Effects of oestradiol and combined norephedrin and oestradiol treatment on female stress incontinence. *Zentralbl Gynaekol* 102: 839,1980.

73 Bergman A, Elia G: Three surgical procedures for genuine stress incontinence: Five-year follow-up of a prospective randomized study. *Am J Obstet Gynecol* 173: 66–71, 1995.

74 Sand PK, Bowen LW, Panganiban R, *et al*.: The low-pressure urethra as a factor in failed retropubic urethropexy. *Obstet Gynecol* 69: 399–401,1987.

75 Beck RP, Grove D, Arnush D, *et al*.: Recurrent urinary stress incontinence treated by the fascia lata sling procedure. *Am J Obstet Gynecol* 120: 613,1974.

76 Horbach NS, Blanco JS, Ostergard DR, *et al.*: A suburethral sling procedure with polytetrafluor-oethylene for the treatment of genuine stress incontinence in patients with low urethral closure pressure. *Obstet Gynecol* 71: 699,1988.

77 Elia G, Bergman A. Genuine stress urinary incontinence with low urethral pressure: 5-year follow-up after Ball-Burch procedure. *J Reprod Med* 40: 503–506,1995.

78 Raz S, Stothers L, Young GP, *et al.*: Vaginal wall sling for anatomical incontinence and intrinsic sphincter dysfunction: Efficacy and outcome analysis. *J Urol* 156: 166–170,1996.

79 McGuire EJ, Appell RA: Transurethral collagen injection for urinary incontinence. *Urology* 43: 413–15,1994.

80 Monga AK, Robinson D, Stanton SL: Perurethral collagen injection for genuine stress inconti-nence: A 2-year follow-up. *Br J Urol* 76: 156–160,1995.

81 Elia G, Bergman A: Ultrasound follow-up of periurethral collagen implant. *Int J Urogyn* in press.

10

Nutritional concerns of menopause

ALESSANDRO LAVIANO AND MICHAEL M MEGUID

Menopause is defined as the final episode of menstrual bleeding in women. However, the term is commonly used to refer to the period of the female climacteric that encompasses the traditional period between the reproductive years up to and beyond the last episode of menstrual bleeding. During this period there is a gradual but progressive loss of ovarian functions, and a variety of endocrine, somatic and psychological changes.

Women approaching menopause are mostly afraid of osteoporosis, breast cancer and coronary heart disease. In prophylaxis against the development of osteoporosis, it is well recognized that a multifaceted approach is sensible: nutrition, exercise and the possible use of estrogen replacement therapy. Certainly, the efficacy of estrogen replacement therapy for osteoporosis prophylaxis has been proven by cross-sectional, longitudinal and retrospective studies.[1]

When women approach the menopause, nevertheless, they are using estrogen replacement therapy as 'intervention therapy,' preventing the natural bone loss that occurs post-menopausally. At the time of the menopausal transition, women present with a bone mass that is a consequence of their lifestyle before the menopause. Peak bone mass occurs at the age of 35 to 40 in White women.[2,3] After that, there is a slight decline in bone mass, followed by an abrupt decline around the time of menopause due to the direct effects of estrogen depletion. Thus estrogen is important in maintaining bone mass postmenopausally and in preventing the decrement in bone mass that leads to fractures immediately after the menopause. Health care professionals, however, need a broader perspective in treating menopausal osteoporosis. A multifaceted prophylactic approach in premenopausal and perimenopausal women should encourage proper nutrition and exercise. In the recent years many studies have investigated different nutritional and exercise modifications that may improve bone mass. We have therefore reviewed those studies, showing how these may add to the advantage of estrogen replacement therapy in decreasing bone loss during menopause. The use of these modalities in lieu of estrogen replacement therapy is also discussed. Nutritional factors that may deal with the prevention of cancer are elaborated on as well, because these are also of major concern to premenopausal and postmenopausal women. It is hoped that this review will allow the physician to deal with the nutritional and lifestyle changes that will contribute to a healthier menopause.

The major nutritional factor that is initially dealt with concerning osteoporosis prophylaxis is the ingestion of calcium and other minerals in the prevention of bone loss. The use of exercise to prevent bone loss in menopausal women is discussed, as well as the limitation of using this as a singular mode for osteoporosis prophylaxis. The nutritional factors that are presented in the section on cancer prevention mainly incorporate a low-fat diet and exercise.

Finally, physicians should clearly try to delineate whether or not patients are using unconventional therapies such as ginseng supplements, acupuncture and others. Because these are outside the usual realm of our medical practice, we tend to ignore these issues. A recent study indicates that 39% of a national survey of 1539 adults used at least one type of unconventional therapy in the last year.[4] There is a paucity of scientific data on the efficacy of such practices. Any attempt to validate suggestions and marketing assertions that ginseng tea and magnesium, for instance, reduce vasomotor symptoms is nonproductive, because there is no double-blind placebo studies determining the efficacy of these alternative therapies. However, physicians should ask about the use of unconventional regimens in their history-taking, and document it in the chart. Without scientific evidence, the current suggestion to patients should be to use all such supplements in moderation. These unconventional regimens, although helpful, should not substitute at the present time for rational, conventional, medical therapy when such is justified (that is, estrogen replacement therapy).

In conclusion, lifestyle habits, nutrition and unconventional medical approaches by our patients are important to be documented in the patient chart, although further scientific knowledge regarding the efficacy and safety of these alternate lifestyle approaches is greatly needed.

OSTEOPOROSIS PROPHYLAXIS

There is a close relationship between estrogen deprivation and the development of osteoporosis. Osteoporosis is one of the dreads of aging. Approximately 25% of aging women and 10% of elderly men experience a vertebral or hip fracture between the age of 60 and 90. Such fractures are a major cause of death and morbidity. Many factors affect the development of osteoporosis, including diet, activity, smoking and general health, and estrogen deprivation is of pivotal importance in this regard.[5] Recently, it has been suggested that the manifestation of osteoporosis in women is influenced to a greater extent by age and years since menopause than by the distribution of nutritional factors in a normal mixed diet.[6]

As outlined by Notelovitz,[7] physicians can play a pivotal role in the screening, prevention and management of osteoporosis by: 1) identifying women with higher risk for osteoporosis at earlier ages; 2) stressing the importance of developing maximal bone mass before menopause; and 3) developing individualized patient prescriptions for bone mass determinants under personal control: exercise, nutrition and hormone replacement therapy.

Estrogen replacement therapy

Optimal bone mass depends on adequate sex hormones, building materials and loading. Sex hormones add to bone mass the amount that is needed for reproduction. When menopause develops, women lose estrogens and their bone mass decreases. It is not known why and which women lose more bone than others and develop osteoporosis. One factor could be latent hypoandrogenism, since even in men the levels of bioavailable testosterone correlate with bone mineral density.[8]

The role of endogenous hormones in preventing bone loss and fractures has been strengthened by a recent study.[9] By measuring serum estradiol concentrations in a large cohort of postmenopausal women, Cummings and colleagues showed that women with undetectable serum estradiol concentrations had a relative risk of 2.5 for subsequent hip or vertebral fracture when compared with women with detectable serum estradiol concentrations. Thus estrogen replacement therapy is the most effective strategy in decreasing bone loss postmenopausally.[1] It is indirectly possible to establish the relative protective effects of exercise in a low-estrogen environment by reviewing studies of young, premenopausal athletes who became amenorrheic. Premenopausal amenorrheic women who are avid exercisers lose bone despite their vigorous exercise activities, but their bone loss may be reversed with estrogen replacement therapy.[10,11] Therefore, exercise in and of itself in a state of estrogen deficiency does not prevent bone loss. An exercise program in combination with estrogen therapy is most beneficial. Proper calcium ingestion and exercise in normal menstruating women will achieve a positive result in improving peak bone mass.

The relative contributions of aging and estrogen deficiency to postmenopausal bone loss have also been studied.[11] Young premature-ovarian-failure patients, perimenopausal patients and postmenopausal patients were studied with bone density measurements at their radial, femoral and lumbar spine sites. It was clear that oophorectomized women who are prematurely menopausal, despite being young in age, had bone densities similar to the nonestrogenized postmenopausal group. They were markedly different from the perimenopausal estrogenized women, who were older and similar in age to the postmenopausal group but had higher bone densities than nonestrogenized younger women.

These studies demonstrate that estrogen deficiency causes bone loss even in young women; if they exercise vigorously and are hypoestrogenemic, they still lose bone.

Exercise

Bones need loading. Mechanoreceptors that transform physical stress into biochemical signals are postulated to exist and to be upregulated by sex hormones. Thus, bone mass increases more after exercise while being exposed to sex hormones (i.e.: premenopausally). The amount of bone mass due to spontaneous activity is likely to be genetically determined.

The effect of exercise on bone mass is site-specific. Therefore, an exercise program that deals mainly with using the lower extremities may improve the femoral neck bone density but may not have any effect on radial bone density. Aerobic exercises, moreover, that improve cardiovascular fitness (walking, swimming) may not be beneficial for bone preservation.[13] However, consistently participating in water exercise appears to be an important factor in preventing bone loss.[14] Thus the appropriate exercise should combine both weight-bearing and aerobic exercise. Aerobic exercise, such as brisk walking, should be done at least two times a week for 20 minutes. Bone density improvement with weights that improve the muscle strength at various upper extremity, lower extremity and spinal sites should also be done for 30 minutes three times a week.[15–17] It is very important to cross-train and not rely on one exercise for both osteoporosis and cardiovascular disease prophylaxis simultaneously. Finally, the exercise is of benefit only if it is continued. Therefore, an exercise program is a program for life.

Prince and colleagues compared the effects of calcium, exercise and estrogen replacement therapy either alone or in combination to prevent bone loss.[18] Data obtained showed that exercise alone improved bone density in women with low bone mass; however, the best results were obtained by the combination of exercise, calcium supplementation and hormone therapy. The specific exercise program was minimal: one weekly exercise class and two brisk 30-minute walks per week. At the exercise classes, the women participated in low-impact aerobic exercise of 1 hour, and 30% of the time was devoted to arm exercise.

Exercise alone has been demonstrated to be effective mainly in the premenopausal period;[19] in this way, peak bone mass attainment is improved before the menopausal transition.[20] A habitual exercise regimen in a normal estrogenic state premenopausally is, therefore, an important determinant in decreasing the propensity for future osteoporosis.[21] However, in the low-estrogen-status women, exercise does not, despite its aerobic benefit, substitute for estrogen replacement therapy, but is an important component in a total health care approach.

Few studies also attempted to show the singular effects of exercise in improving bone density in postmenopausal women. Because these are short-term studies, it is impossible to ascertain if there is a lasting effect on bone density. The effects of exercise in osteoporotic women with vigorous loading exercises demonstrated an increase in bone mass of 3.8%, whereas the controls demonstrated bone loss by 1.9%.[15–17] Another study looked at maximum oxygen uptakes to test the improvement in aerobic capacity and then studied, via neutron activator analysis, the total body calcium level of women at a level of physical activity that improved the maximum oxygen intake. An increase in the amount of calcium stored in bone was found. Positive results (average increases of 6% in lumbar bone density and 1.4% in density of the radius) were also noted in individuals using more diverse exercise programs, such as aerobics, calistenics and stair climbing. Finally, Notelovitz investigated the effect of estrogen replacement therapy and exercise with a resistance circuit weight training program.[22] The greatest increase in spinal density (9.4%) was found in the group receiving estrogen replacement therapy and physically exercising.

These positive results must not lead us to underestimate the evidence that when exercise, calcium and estrogen replacement therapy are compared, estrogen replacement therapy is the most beneficial.

Nutritional factors

Calcium and vitamin D are most important contributors to bone mass. Osteoporotics absorb less calcium from the gut than controls, probably because of unfavorable gene alleles for the vitamin D receptor. Furthermore, the general supply of calcium and vitamin D in the normal population could be of greater significance than assumed. The combination of a receptor defect and a latent deficiency could be deleterious.

CALCIUM

The elemental calcium RDA is 1 g for premenopausal women and 1.5 g for nonestrogenized postmenopausal women.[23] More recently, Weaver attempted to estimate average calcium requirements for various age groups by gender.[24] Surprisingly, these estimates exceed the current RDA for females aged six to 16 years and older than 30 years and for men aged six to 30 years. They also exceed current calcium intakes in the US during adolescence for both sexes and for females above the age of 11. These data suggest that a latent calcium deficiency could be present in the population.

Calcium is a threshold nutrient, which means that a nutritional response in terms of calcium balance or bone mass will be present at intakes below the threshold and not above.

As Dawson-Hughes and colleagues have shown in the postmenopausal woman, there is a critical level of calcium that is necessary to maintain bone mass.[25] Healthy postmenopausal women with a daily calcium intake less than 400 mg significantly reduced bone loss by increasing their calcium intake to at least 800 mg per day. Calcium citrate maleate was more effective at all bone sites than calcium carbonate because of a better bioavailability, although calcium carbonate is more readily available and is less expensive. Calcium citrate maleate is better absorbed but is more expensive, and most elderly patients may have achlorhydria, which prevents the absorption of calcium carbonate from the gastrointestinal tract.[26] Also, there is a well-defined enhancing effect of the coingestion of a meal with calcium supplements. It would seem prudent to recommend that any calcium supplement be given at meal times.[27]

In the postmenopausal woman, calcium as a therapy is not as effective as estrogen replacement therapy, but it reduces bone mass in individuals who ingest less than 400 mg per day of calcium. As recently shown by Fardellone and colleagues,[28] calcium supplementation is effective in reducing markers of bone turnover (hydroxyproline, pyridinoline, and deoxypyridinoline) in postmenopausal women, with a greater effect in women with a low dietary calcium intake. Dietary calcium also appears to have an impact on hip fracture risk.[29] The results of a follow-up study involving a cohort of 4342 white men and postmenopausal women aged 50 to 74 years show that, although not statistically significant, the age-adjustment risk of hip fracture was approximately 50% lower in the highest quartile of calcium intake compared with the lowest quartile in the subgroup of women who were at least six years postmenopausal and not taking postmenopausal hormones.

In conclusion, detailing a calcium intake history is extremely important: if calcium intake falls below a critical level, namely 400 mg per day, substitutive therapy in the form of pills to increase calcium intake to at least 800 mg per day has proven beneficial.

Calcium nutrition is most important during growth and development to achieve genetically determined peak skeletal mass in premenopausal women.[30,31] Therefore, calcium intake seems to have its greatest impact in premenopausal women. Matkovite and colleagues detailed bone status and fracture rates in two different regions of Yugoslavia with very different calcium ingestions.[32] In one district, the daily calcium intake was twice that in another district. The group with the higher calcium intake had, throughout their lifetimes (both in the male and female population), a lower risk of fracture at all bone sites. A three-year prospective study in premenopausal women showed that increasing dietary calcium intake by an average of 610 mg per day improved lumbar bone density.[33] Also calcium supplementation in pill form in perimenopausal women has been proved to improve lumbar bone density.[34] Finally, a study in a homogeneous population of French-Canadian women showed that one of the major variables in terms of subsequent bone mass was calcium intake in early adulthood.[3] Therefore, physicians should make sure calcium intake is above a certain critical level. They should also consider this issue important in premenopausal patients. The main benefit of calcium is to improve peak bone mass. In the postmenopausal woman it is adjunct but not a substitute for estrogen replacement therapy.

VITAMIN D

Vitamin D regulates bone mineral homeostasis by increasing serum levels of calcium and phosphate, principally by stimulating intestinal calcium and phosphate absorption. Estrogen administration to postmenopausal women raises the serum levels of the active metabolite of vitamin D, $1,25(OH)_2D$, presumably through increased renal production, and this increase is associated with enhanced intestinal calcium transport. Although reduced intestinal calcium absorption has been reported in postmenopausal women, there is no consistent evidence of a decrease of 1,25(OH)$_2$D at the time of menopause. Thus some investigators have addressed the issue of tissue resistance to 1,25(OH)$_2$D. Recent data from Krall and colleagues show that the genotype of the 1,25(OH)$_2$D receptor (VDR) influences bone accretion or loss.[35] The VDR genotype was determined in 229 healthy postmenopausal women, and VDR alleles were designated according to the presence (b) or absence (B) of the BsmI restriction enzyme cutting site. The results showed that among women more than 10 years postmenopausal, those with the BB genotype had the lowest femoral neck bone mineral density. Furthermore, rates of bone loss over two years were greater in the BB group. These data clearly indicate that a genetic susceptibility exists in predisposing to osteoporosis. This hypothesis has recently been supported by Deng and colleagues,[36] who showed that change of bone mass in postmenopausal women is associated with VDR and estrogen receptor genotypes.

Clinical trials with vitamin D show promise.[37] Excesses of vitamin D are important to avoid because hypervitaminosis of vitamin D can cause hypercalcemia and hypercalciuria, leading to nephrolithiasis and/or nephrocalcinosis. Vitamin D treatment will probably prove most efficacious in populations with marginal vitamin D intake and/or limited sunlight exposure. It has been demonstrated that bone mass increases during the period June to December and decreases during the period December to June.[38] Moreover, Dawson-Hughes and colleagues showed that in climates where there is a lack of sunlight, bone density falls in postmenopausal women.[39] In healthy postmenopausal women in northern climates, vitamin D intakes of 500 IU during the 'sunless' season can significantly reduce late-wintertime bone loss and improve net bone density of the spine. Therefore, it appears that the need for vitamin D may vary according to the season, but this may be geographically determined.

FLUORIDE

Fluoride supplementation has also been suggested for the treatment of bone loss. Initially, fluoride showed promise because of an increase in trabecular bone density.[40–42] Unfortunately, subsequent results have been disappointing, because similar positive effects of fluoride were not observed on cortical bone mass. The bone formed is also more fragile. Fluoride can also create lower-extremity pain syndromes and gastric irritation. Thus it is not recommended as a supplement for osteoporosis prophylaxis.

ZINC

In osteoporotic individuals, zinc excretion level is higher than in nonosteoporotic individuals,[43] probably secondary to increased bone resorption. High zinc excretion also occurs in hypermetabolic states such as surgery, burns, alcoholic cirrhosis, thalassemia and starvation; in patients on total parenteral nutrition, and in various conditions of hormonal disturbances that cause bone loss, that is, hyperparathyroidism, thyrotoxicosis, and Cushing's disease. Zinc is also excreted in sweat, so that after vigorous exercise, zinc loss occurs. Currently, there are no dietary recommendations for using zinc as a prophylaxis agent against osteoporosis. The RDA for zinc is 15 mg per day.

BORON AND MAGNESIUM

Deficiencies in boron and magnesium can affect the formation and maintenance of bones[44] and thus the development of osteoporosis. There also seems to be a relationship between boron and magnesium; their combined effect modifies calcium metabolism and bone density. Animal studies indicate that magnesium deprivation creates a need for boron to equilibrate calcium metabolism. The levels of magnesium and of boron per day in these studies fluctuated between 115 and 315 mg per day, and 0.23 and 3.23 mg per day, respectively. The absolute RDA requirements for boron and magnesium in postmenopausal women have not been established. Further information is needed regarding this issue because it is possible that calcium supplementation may require these minerals to become effective as a dietary supplement.[44]

In conclusion, osteoporosis affects one in four women over the age of 65. Intervention can reduce bone loss at any point and perhaps increase bone density, but no known therapy can restore the normal bone architecture once it is lost.[45] Cross-sectional and longitudinal studies indicate that calcium supplementation in postmenopausal women is important despite the overshadowing positive effect of estrogen replacement therapy on bone density. Women who have low intakes of calcium (less than 400 mg per day) improve their bone density by increasing their intake to 800 mg per day. Calcium citrate maleate may be the preferred supplement, although calcium carbonate may be substituted because of the ease of availability and lower cost. Fluoride is not beneficial. The need for zinc, boron and magnesium supplements awaits further documentation before we prescribe these clinically. Finally, the need for extra vitamin D may be seasonal and geographic, and probably most efficacious in populations with marginal vitamin D intake.

Effects of adverse lifestyle choices on bone loss

SMOKING

A connection between calcium-deficient nutrition and other unhealthy lifestyles, such as lack of exercise, smoking and regular alcohol intake, has been shown by multivariate analysis.[46] Smoking and the by-products of nicotinic acid have an effect on ovarian function[47] and even change the metabolic clearance rate of exogenous hormones.[48] Furthermore, smoking has an impact on the age of menopause.[49] The mean age of menopause is 51.4 plus or minus 1.19 years. Curiously, there has been no secular trend toward a later age of menopause in the last 25 years. Smokers reach menopause at an average age of 1.74 years earlier than nonsmokers. They therefore go through the changes of estrogen deprivation sooner and also tend to be slimmer and have less body fat.[50,51] The slender smoker has a greater risk for osteoporosis. It is also suggested that smoking is associated with a decrease in calcium absorption. It is difficult to attribute a singular effect of smoking on bone density, because smokers ingest a higher level of caffeine and generally consume more alcohol.[51] However, controlling for caffeine intake and alcohol, smokers still have much lower bone densities than nonsmokers; smoking again appears to affect calcium absorption through the gastrointestinal tract. Smoking, therefore, causes an earlier menopause, increases the clearance of exogenous sex steroid hormones, is associated with thinner stature, and may decrease calcium absorption through the gastrointestinal tract. All of these effects cause a decrease in bone mass.

ALCOHOL

It is clearly known that alcoholics have a higher incidence of bone fractures, some of which may be explained by an increased exposure to trauma when they are inebriated; however, the possible increase in fractures in alcoholics may also be secondary to bone fragility. Studies have shown that, in looking at bone density at five skeletal sites, the mean annual loss of bone minerals in alcoholics is 2% higher than that of controls.[52] Animals fed ethanol diets have been shown to have lower bone densities as compared with controls. A possible factor contributing to bone loss in alcoholics is an impairment in vitamin D metabolism due to liver cirrhosis. Alcoholics who develop peptic ulcers may also have problems with absorption of nutrients.

Some of the difficulty with alcohol-related studies is that the reporting of such is subject to shame. It has been assessed that approximately 50% to 70% of postmenopausal women report the use of alcohol. It is difficult to state what the relationship would be between peripheral estradiol levels and excessive alcohol consumption. In one study, estradiol levels appear to be increased in alcoholic women, but this doesn't seem to be associated with lower bone density.[53] Further work on nutrient absorption in alcoholics and the effect on endogenous and exogenous sex hormones is needed.

LACTOSE MALABSORPTION

Despite of the emphasis on increasing calcium absorption through the diet, physicians should make sure to avoid prescribing such a diet to lactose-intolerant individuals. In a study done in New Zealand, lactose malabsorption was assessed by measuring breath hydrogen after a 50 g oral lactose tolerance test.[54] A highest prevalence of lactose malabsorption in hip fractures cases was observed. Sixty per cent of elderly hip fracture patients were lactose malabsorbers compared with 12% of young controls, whereas other reports had stated that 27% to 65% of osteoporotic populations and 10% to 15% of healthy control populations were lactose intolerant. Decreased dietary calcium intake, not poor calcium absorption, is believed to augment osteoporotic bone loss in lactose malabsorbers. Low dietary calcium intake would then result in lower peak bone mass attainment. Milk seems to be the most irritating factor in lactose malabsorbers, whereas cheese and yogurt are better tolerated and thus seem to be a better source of calcium. In these individuals, dietary supplementation with calcium pills is appropriate.

VEGETARIAN DIETS

Vegetarian diets may have an impact on peripheral estrogen levels. Goldin and colleagues studied 10 vegetarian and 10 nonvegetarian premenopausal women on four occasions approximately four months apart.[55] They found that vegetarians consumed less total fat than omnivores and they also consumed more dietary fiber. In both groups they measured urinary and fecal excretion of estrogen, and found that vegetarian women had an increased fecal output, which in turn led to an increased fecal excretion of estrogen and decreased plasma concentration of estrogen. The implications for this are complex, since the higher excretion rate of estrogen may in fact promote osteoporosis, which this study did not specifically detail. A low-fat diet, however, has been associated with a lower risk of heart disease. Although this is of great interest, the dietary effect of a vegetarian diet on bone metabolism needs to be further elucidated.

An intriguing issue is the role of dietary protein intake in osteoporosis. By analysing 104,338 person-years (the number of subjects studied times the number of years of follow-up), Munger and colleagues[56] have recently demonstrated that intake of dietary protein, especially from animal sources, may be associated with a reduced incidence of hip fractures in postmenopausal women.

CAFFEINE

Excess caffeine intake is associated with osteoporosis. In a large field study involving 205 healthy, nonsmoking, postmenopausal women, the effects of caffeine consumption on rates of change in bone mineral density were investigated.[57] The results obtained show that daily consumption of caffeine in amounts equal to or greater than that obtained from about two or three servings of brewed coffee may accelerate bone loss from the spine and total body in women with calcium intakes below the recommended dietary allowance of 800 mg per day. Because skeletal mass represents the cumulative effects of genetic and environmental lifestyle factors, issues such as common dietary intake of caffeine should also be taken into account when promoting an osteoporosis prophylaxis program.

CORONARY HEART DISEASE PROPHYLAXIS

The Framingham Study was the first to detail the physiologic changes that occur in women postmenopausally and their relationship to lipid profile changes and cardiovascular disease incidence.[58–60] Women seem to lag behind men in incidence of coronary heart disease by 10 years. It is, however, a leading cause of death in postmenopausal women. There are a number of different factors that may make this possible in the postmenopausal period.

Blood lipids

According to the Framingham Study, high-density lipoprotein (HDL) cholesterol remains stable postmenopausally and is always higher in women than in men of similar age groups.[61] Low-density lipoprotein (LDL) cholesterol rises in the postmenopausal age group, probably because of a reduced activity of LDL receptors.[62] Thus, a shift in the HDL to LDL cholesterol ratio occurs. The total to HDL cholesterol ratio estimates are therefore important in evaluating for risk of heart disease. When this ratio exceeds 7.5, women have the same cardiovascular heart disease risk as men. In addition, postmenopausal women have higher levels of lipoprotein(a), an atherogenic particle that has been shown to be an important independent risk factor for coronary heart disease.[63] Finally, estrogen replacement therapy may negatively affect blood lipids especially in dyslipidemic women, thus increasing the possibility of coronary heart disease occurrence.[64] Fortunately, this risk appears to be reduced by newer hormonal therapies.[65]

To reduce the risk of coronary heart disease in postmenopausal women, particularly in dyslipidemic patients, a low-fat high-fiber diet is recommended.[66,67] However, it must be remembered that dairy products contribute a considerable proportion of the fat intake, and are thus often reduced. Unfortunately, dairy products provide approximately 60% of dietary calcium. Therefore, specific advice about calcium should be given to women commencing lipid-lowering diets, in order to attain recommended intakes and to reduce the risk of osteoporosis as well as coronary heart disease.[68]

Myocardial infarction

Unrecognized myocardial infarctions are particularly significant problems for women, who would benefit from closer periodic electrocardiogram surveillance and more attention to atypical symptoms of heart attack presentation. Black women seem to have the poorest prognosis after myocardial infarction.[69] The cumulative mortality of 48 months for heart attacks in all women was 36% versus 21% for men. The cumulative mortality, however, by race was 34% for Blacks versus 24% for Whites. The poor prognosis for women was influenced by a particularly higher mortality rate among Black women: 48%. The mortality rate for White women was 32%, for Black men 23%, and for White men 21%.

Fat distribution may also play a role in the increased cardiovascular risk of postmenopausal women. In a recent review, Tchernof and colleagues[70] suggest that part of the increased incidence of cardiovascular disease in postmenopausal women may be attributable to increased central body fatness, and that therapies aiming at preventing these changes in fat distribution such as hormone replacement therapy, diet or exercise are likely to provide long-term cardiovascular and metabolic benefits for women's health. An interesting new approach to coronary heart disease prevention has been addressed by Bostick and colleagues.[71] By studying a prospective cohort of 34,486 postmenopausal women during more than 10 years, they tried to ascertain whether greater intakes of calcium, vitamin D or milk products may protect against ischemic heart disease mortality. Results obtained suggest that a higher intake of calcium, but not of vitamin D or milk products, is associated with reduced cardiovascular mortality in postmenopausal women, and reduced risk may be achievable whether the high intake of calcium is attained by diet, supplements, or both.

Diabetes

Women are particularly vulnerable to the cardiovascular sequelae of diabetes. Diabetes increases cardiovascular disease risk threefold in women and puts them at the same risk as men of the same age. In a separate Framingham analysis, the effect of diabetes doubled the risk of recurrent myocardial infarction in women – a relative risk of 2.1 – but had an insignificant effect on men.[72] An increased susceptibility to cardiac failure among diabetic women was an important factor in determining survivorship. Women with diabetes developed cardiac failure four times more often (16%) than women without diabetes, in which the rate of occurrence of cardiac failure was 3.8%. The increased propensity in diabetic women still needs to be better investigated. However, it is thought that the toxic effects of poorly controlled diabetes have a more damaging effect on the female myocardium. Furthermore, when cardiac failure developed, 25% of diabetic women experienced a recurrent myocardial infarction or fatal coronary event, more than doubling the rate when diabetes was absent. In conclusion, a diabetic Black woman is at highest risk for dying of a myocardial infarction. Careful evaluation of such high-risk individuals is mandatory so that a myocardial infaraction is not missed. Diabetic diets and control of blood glucose by proper diet is of vital importance.

OBESITY

Another major contributing factor to heart disease incidence appears to be obesity. The results of the Nurses' Health Study show that even mild to moderate overweight in middle-aged individuals increases the risk for coronary heart disease.[73] Further studies suggested that, besides the overall quantity of excess fat, the pattern of body fat distribution is important.[74] The deposition of fat predominantly in the abdomen and upper body has been associated with high blood pressure, glucose intolerance, and dyslipidemia.

Finally, aerobic conditioning exercise is an important element in preventing heart disease. Low-dose aspirin therapy is also used. However, despite our advice to women to use these modalities, most of the studies indicating efficacy of aspirin and exercise have been in men.

BREAST CANCER PROPHYLAXIS

Aside from the issues of coronary heart disease incidence in women and lifestyle and body fat intake changes, the implications that diet may have on an increased risk for breast cancer are also important. The dominant protective factors against the development of breast cancer, however, seem to be genetic. Women who have a strong family history, namely, a mother and a sister who have had breast cancer, have a relative risk of 14 of developing breast cancer.[75] A clear relationship exists between breast cancer and estrogen, since the length of estrogenicity of the individual – that is, early menarche, late menopause, decreased, delayed or no childbearing with recurrent increased numbers of ovulatory cycles – may increase the propensity of breast cancer. Also, early surgical menopause, that is before the age 35, seems to have a protective effect, reducing the relative risk of breast cancer to 0.6 compared with women who have gone through natural menopause. It is, therefore, hard to delineate the very controversial association between estrogenicity and breast cancer and to isolate dietary factors that may have a role in promoting breast cancer rates.

An important issue in the prevention of breast cancer is the role of dietary fat. The current opinion is that high fat intake, in particular of animal fat, is a primary cause of breast cancer in different countries. However, as Willett outlined in his review, all the studies to date have not definitely shown a protective effect against breast cancer by decreasing dietary fat to less than 30% of the daily diet.[76] Also, the Nurses' Health Study showed that moderate reduction of fat intake by adult women is unlikely to result in a substantial reduction in the incidence of breast cancer.[73] On the other hand, analysis of postmenopausal women in Hawaii estimated that 10% to 20% of breast cancer could be prevented by notably decreasing saturated fat intake.[77] Thus the association between dietary fat and breast cancer is difficult to validate objectively, probably because of the difficulty of collecting accurate dietary information and other methodologic limitations. However, it appears safe to recommend to perimenopausal women a low-fat, high-fiber diet, which significantly reduces estradiol and estrone levels without affecting ovulation.[78] Also, the management of localized breast cancer may be positively influenced by adjuvant fat intake reduction.[79]

Anthropomorphic changes in fat distribution may have an association with breast cancer risk.[80–82] Patients with breast cancer have a significantly greater waist to hip circumference ratio than controls. Although obese women have been associated with a higher risk of breast cancer, it is felt that women in whom fat distribution is of android type, constitute a subgroup of obese women who appear to be at significantly highest risk of developing breast cancer. Also, obese women who develop breast cancer tend to have more axillary node involvement than their leaner counterparts. The confounding factor here may be that obese women may present with locally advanced breast cancer more often than their leaner counterparts because their body and breast size may result in a delay in detecting the tumor. Recent data also suggest that the timing of weight gain may be related to breast cancer risk. Kumar and colleagues found that women who progressively gain weight from puberty to adulthood, and specifically in the third decade of life, should be considered at a higher risk for developing breast cancer.[83] Excessive weight gain in women at the time of intense hormonal change can result in metabolic dysfunction, while the susceptibility of mammary tissue to carcinogenesis is greatest in early adult life. Thus excessive weight gain in that age group is associated with the development of hyperinsulinemia in individuals with genetic susceptibility to insulin resistance. Hence insulin resistance syndrome may be a metabolic link between weight gain and breast cancer risk.[84]

Finally, the increase in the risk or breast cancer associated with a high waist to hip ratio, low parity or greater age at first pregnancy is more pronounced among women with a family history of breast cancer. Other factors that may affect the development of breast cancer and that may indirectly be associated with changes in diet are exercise and alcohol intake. Vigorous exercise may actually decrease the lifetime occurrence of all cancers.[85] Excess alcohol ingestion alone increases breast cancer rates to 1.6,[76] and this issue may confound studies purporting to show a slight increase in breast cancer rates with exogenous sex steroid hormone therapy.[86]

REFERENCES

1 Ravnikar VA: Hormonal management of osteoporosis. *Clin Obstet Gynecol* 35: 913–922,1992.

2 Bonjour J-P, Theintz G, Buchs B, *et al.*: Critical years and stages of puberty for spinal and femoral bone mass accumulation during adolescence. *J Clin Endocrinol Metab* 73: 555–563,1992.

3 Picard D, Ste-Marie LG, Coutu D, *et al.*: Premenopausal bone mineral content relates to height, weight and calcium intake during early adulthood. *Bone Miner* 4: 299–309,1988.

4 Eisenberg DM, Kessler RC, Foster C, *et al.*: Unconventional medicine in the United States: Prevalence, cost, and patterns of use. *N Engl J Med* 328: 246–252,1993.

5 Christiansen C: Osteoporosis: Diagnosis and management today and tomorrow. *Bone* 17 (suppl 5): 513S–516s,1995.

6 Preisinger E, Leitner G, Uher E, *et al.*: Nutrition and osteoporosis: A nutritional analysis of women in postmenopause. *Wien Klin Wochenschr* 107: 418–422,1995.

7 Notelovitz M: Osteoporosis: Screening, prevention and management. *Fertil Steril* 59: 707–725,1993.

8 Ziegler R, Scheidt-Nave C, Scharla S: Pathophysiology of osteoporosis: Unresolved problems and new insights. J Nutr 125 (suppl 7): 2033S–2037S, 1995.

9 Cummings SR, Browner WS, Bauer D, *et al.*: Endogenous hormones and the risk of hip and vertebral fractures among older women. Study of osteoporotic fractures research group. *N Engl Med* 339: 733–738,1998.

10 Drinkwater BL, Nilson K, Chestnut CH, *et al.*: Bone mineral content of amenorrheic and menorrheic athletes. *N Engl J Med* 311: 277–281,1984.

11 Drinkwater BL, Nilson K, Att S, *et al.*: Bone mineral density after resumption of menses in amenorrheic women. *JAMA* 256: 380–382,1986.

12 Richelson LS, Wahner HW, Melton LJ III, *et al.*: Relative contributions of aging and estrogen deficiency to postmenopausal bone loss. *N Engl J Med* 311: 1273–1275,1984.

13 Cavanaugh DJ, Cann CE: Brisk walking does not stop bone loss in postmenopausal women. *Bone* 9: 201–204,1988.

14 Tsukahara N, Toda A, Goto J, Ezawa L: Cross–sectional and longitudinal studies on the effect of water exercise in controlling bone loss in Japanese postmenopausal women. *J Nutr Sci Vitaminol Tokyo* 40: 37–47,1994.

15 Chow RK, Harrison JE, Brown CF, *et al.*: Physical fitness effect on bone mass in postmenopausal women. *Arch Phys Med Rehabil* 67: 231–234,1986.

16 Simkin A, Ayalon J, Leichter I: Increased trabecular bone density due to bone-loading exercises in postmenopausal osteoporotic women. *Calcif Tissue Int* 40: 59–63,1987.

17 Smith EL, Smith PE, Ensign CJ, *et al.*: Bone involution decrease in exercising middle-aged women. *Calcif Tissue Int* 36: S129–S138,1984.

18 Prince RL, Smith M, Dick IM, *et al.*: Prevention of postmenopausal osteoporosis. A comparative

study of exercise, calcium supplementation, and hormone-replacement therapy. *N Engl J Med* 325: 1189–1195,1991.

19 Bassey EJ, Rothwell MC, Littlewood JJ, Pye DW: Pre- and postmenopausal women have different bone mineral density responses to the same high-impact exercises. *J Bone Miner Res* 13: 1805–1813,1998.

20 Aloia JF, Vaswani AN, Yeh JK, *et al.*: Premenopausal bone mass is related to physical activity. *Arch Intern Med* 148: 121–123,1988.

21 Stevenson JC, Lees B, Devenport M, *et al.*: Determinants of bone density in normal women, risk factors for future osteoporosis? *Br Med J* 298: 924–928,1989.

22 Notelovitz M: Exercise and health maintenance in menopausal women. *Ann NY Acad Sci* 592: 204–220,1990.

23 Dawson-Hughes B: Calcium supplementation and bone loss: A review of controlled clinical trials. *Am J Clin Nutr* 54: 274S–280S,1991.

24 Weaver CM: Age-related calcium requirements due to changes in absorption and utilization. *J Nutr* 124 (Suppl 8): 1418S–1425S,1994.

25 Dawson-Hughes B, Dallal GE, Krall EA, *et al.*: A controlled trial of the effect of calcium supplementation on bone density in postmenopausal women. *N Engl J Med* 323: 878–883,1990.

26 Recker RR: Calcium absorption and achlorhydria. *N Engl J Med* 313: 70–73,1985.

27 Recker RR: Prevention of osteoporosis: Calcium nutrition. *Osteoporos Int* 3 (Suppl 1): 163–165,1993.

28 Fardellone P, Brazier M, Kamel S, *et al.*: Biochemical effects of calcium supplementation in postmenopausal women: influence of dietary calcium intake. *Am J Clin Nutr* 67: 1273–1278,1998.

29 Looker AC, Harris TB, Madans JH, Sempos CT: Dietary calcium and hip fracture risk: The NHANES I Epidemiologic Follow-Up Study. *Osteoporos Int* 3: 177–184,1993.

30 Lindsay R, Nieves J, Golden A, Kelsey J: Bone mass among premenopausal women. *Int J Fertil Menopausal Stud* 38 (Suppl 2): 83–87,1993.

31 Baran DT: Magnitude and determinants of premenopausal bone loss. *Osteoporos Int* 4 (Suppl 1): 31–34,1994.

32 Matkovic V, Kostial K, Simonovic I, *et al.*: Bone status and fracture rates in two regions of Yugoslavia. *Am J Clin Nutr* 32: 540–549,1979.

33 Baran D, Sorensen A, Grimes J, *et al.*: Dietary modification with diary products for preventing vertebral bone loss in premenopausal women: A three-year prospective study. *J Clin Endocrinol Metab* 70: 264–270,1990.

34 Elders PJM, Netelenbos JC, Lips P, *et al.*: Calcium supplementation reduces vertebral bone loss in perimenopausal women: A controlled trial in 248 women between 46 and 55 years of age. *J Clin Endocrinol Metab* 73: 533–540,1991.

35 Krall EA, Parry P, Lichter JB, Dawson-Hughes B: Vitamin D receptor alleles and rates of bone loss: Influences of years since menopause and calcium intake. *J Bone Miner Res* 10: 978–984,1995.

36 Deng HW, Li J, Li JL, *et al.*: Change of bone mass in postmenopausal women with and without hormone replacement therapy is associated with vitamin D receptor and estrogen receptor genotypes. *Hum Genet* 103: 576–585,1998.

37 Bikle DD: Role of vitamin D, its metabolites, and analogs in the management of osteoporosis. *Rheum Dis Clin North Am* 20: 759–775,1994.

38 Dawson-Hughes B, Harris S: Regional changes in body composition by time of year in healthy postmenopausal women. *Am J Clin Nutr* 56: 307–313,1992.

39 Dawson–Hughes B, Dallal GE, Krall EA, *et al.*: Effect of vitamin D supplementation on wintertime and overall bone loss in healthy postmenopausal women. *Ann Intern Med* 115: 505–512,1991.

40 Farley SM, Libanati CR, Odvina CV, *et al.*: Efficacy of long-term fluoride and calciumtherapy in correcting the deficit of spinal bone density in osteoporosis. *J Clin Epidemiol* 42: 1067–1074,1989.

41 Liote F, Bardin C, Liou A, *et al.*: Bioavailability of fluoride in postmenopausal women: compara-

tive study between sodium fluoride and disodium monofluorophosphate-calcium carbonate. *Calcif Tissue Int* 50: 209–213,1992.

42 Riggs BL, Hodgson SF, O'Fallon WM, *et al*.: Effect of fluoride treatment on the fracture rate in postmenopausal women with osteoporosis. *N Engl J Med* 322: 802–809,1990.

43 Herzberg M, Foldes J, Steinberg R, *et al*.: Zinc excretion in osteoporotic women. *J Bone Miner Res* 5: 251–257,1990.

44 Nielsen FH: Studies on the relationship between boron and magnesium which possibly affects the formation and maintenance of bones. *Magnes Trace Elem* 9: 61–69,1990.

45 Licata AA: Prevention and osteoporosis management. *Cleve Clin J Med* 61: 451–460,1994.

46 Gass RR, Gutzwiller F: Epidemiology of osteoporosis. *Schweiz Rundson Med Prax* 81: 1395–1400,1992.

47 Friedman AJ, Ravnikar V, Barbieri RL, *et al*.: Serum steroid hormone profiles in postmenopausal smokers and nonsmokers. *Fertil Steril* 47: 398–401,1987.

48 Jensen J, Christiansen C, Rodbro P: Cigarette smoking, serum estrogens, and bone loss during hormone replacement therapy early after menopause. *N Engl J Med* 313: 973–975,1985.

49 McKinlay SM, Bifano NL, McKinlay JB: Smoking and age at menopause in women. *Ann Intern Med* 103: 350–356,1985.

50 Daniell HW: Osteoporosis of the slender smoker. Vertebral compression fractures and loss of metacarpal cortex in relation to postmenopausal cigarette smoking and lack of obesity. *Arch Intern Med* 136: 298–304,1976.

51 Krall EA, Dawon-Hughes B: Smoking and bone loss among postmenopausal women. *J Bone Miner Res* 6: 331–338,1991.

52 Dalen N, Lamke B: Bone mineral losses in alcoholics. *Acta Orthop Scand* 47: 469–471,1976.

53 Gavalier JS, Love K: Detection of the relationship between moderate alcoholic beverage consumption and serum levels of estradiol in normal postmenopausal women: Effects of alcohol consumption, quantitation methods and sample size adequacy. *J Stud Alcohol* 53: 389–394,1992.

54 Wheadon M, Goulding A, Barbezat GO, *et al*.: Lactose malabsorption and calcium intake as risk factors for osteoporosis in elderly New Zealand women. *NZ Med J* 104: 417–419,1991.

55 Goldin BR, Adlercreutz H, Gorbach SL, *et al*.: Estrogen excretion patterns and plasma levels in vegetarian and omnivorous women. *N Engl J Med* 307: 1542–1547,1982.

56 Munger RD, Cerhan JR, Chiu BC: Prospective study of dietary protein intake and risk of hip fracture in postmenopausal women. *Am J Clin Nutr* 69: 147–152,1999.

57 Harris SS, Dawson-Hughes B: Caffeine and bone loss in healthy postmenopausal women. *Am J Clin Nutr* 60: 573–578,1994.

58 Kannel WB: Metabolic risk factors for coronary heart disease in women: Perspective from the Framingham Study. *Am Heart J* 114: 413–419,1987.

59 Lerner DJ, Kannel WB: Patterns of coronary heart disease morbidity and mortality in the sexes: A 26-year follow-up of the Framingham population. *Am Heart J* 113: 383–309,1986.

60 Matthews KA, Meilahn E, Kuller LH, *et al*.: Menopause and risk factors for coronary heart disease. *N Engl J Med* 322: 882–889,1990.

61 Van Beresteijn EC, Korevaar JC, Huijbregts PC, *et al*.: Perimenopausal increase in serum cholesterol: A 10-year longitudinal study. *Am J Epidemiol* 137: 383–392,1993.

62 Arca M, Vega GL, Grundy SM: Hypercholesterolemia in postmenopausal women. Metabolic defects and response to low-dose lovastatin. *JAMA* 271: 453–459,1994.

63 Jenner JL, Ordovas JM, Lamon-Fava S, *et al*.: Effects of age, sex, and menopausal status on plasma lipoprotein(a) levels. The Framingham Offspring Study. *Circulation* 87: 1135–1141,1993.

64 Granfone A, Campos H, McNamara JR, *et al*.: Effects of estrogen replacement on plasma lipoproteins and apolipoproteins in postmenopausal, dyslipidemic women. *Metabolism* 41: 1193–1198,1992.

65 Conrad J, Basdevant A, Thomas JL, *et al.*: Cardiovascular risk factors and combined estrogen–progestin replacement therapy: A placebo-controlled study with nomegestrol acetate and estradiol. *Fertil Steril* 64: 957–962,1995.

66 Jacques H, Noreau L, Moorjani S. Effects on plasma lipoproteins and endogenous sex hormones of substituting lean white fish for other animal-protein sources in diets of postmenopausal women. *Am J Clin Nutr* 55: 896–901,1992.

67 Maruyama C, Nakamura M, Ito M, Ezawa I: The effect of milk and skim milk intake on serum lipids and apoproteins in postmenopausal females. *J Nutr Sci Vitaminol Tokyo* 38: 203–213,1992.

68 Walker J, Ball M: Increasing calcium intake in women on a low-fat diet. *Eur J Clin Nutr* 47: 718–723,1993.

69 Tofler GH, Stone PH, Muller JE, *et al.*: Effects of gender and race on prognosis after myocardial infarction: Adverse prognosis for women, particularly black women. *J Am Coll Cardiol* 9: 473–482,1987.

70 Tchernof A, Calles-Escandon J, Sites CK, Poehlman ET: Menopause, central body fatness, and insulin resistance: effects of hormone replacement therapy. *Coron Artery Dis* 9: 503–511,1998.

71 Bostick RM, Kushi LH, Wu Y, *et al.*: Relation of calcium, vitamin D, and dairy food intake to ischemic heart disease mortality among postmenopausal women. *Am J Epidemiol* 149: 151–161,1999.

72 Abbott RD, Donahue RP, Kannel WB, *et al.*: The impact of diabetes on survival following myocardial infarction in men vs women. The Framingham Study. *JAMA* 260: 3456–3460,1988.

73 Willett WC, Stampfer MJ, Colditz GA, *et al.*: Dietary fat and the risk of breast cancer. *N Engl J Med* 316: 22–28,1987.

74 Despres J-P, Moorjani S, Lupien PJ, *et al.*: Regional distribution of body fat, plasma lipoproteins, and cardiovascular disease. *Arteriosclerosis* 10: 497–511,1990.

75 Sattin RW, Rubin GL, Webster LA, *et al.*: Family history and the risk of breast cancer. *JAMA* 253: 1908–1913,1985.

76 Willett WC: The search for the causes of breast and colon cancer. *Nature* 338: 389–394,1989.

77 Hankin JH: Role of nutrition in women's health: Diet and breast cancer. *J Am Diet Assoc* 93: 994–999,1993.

78 Bagga D, Ashley JM, Geffrey SP, *et al.*: Effects of a very low-fat, high-fiber diet on serum hormones and menstrual function. Implications for breast cancer prevention. *Cancer* 76: 2491–2496,1995.

79 Chlebowski RT, Rose D, Buzzard IM, *et al.*: Adjuvant dietary fat intake reduction in postmenopausal breast cancer patient management. The Women's Intervention Nutrition Study (WINS). *Breast Cancer Res Treat* 20: 73–84,1992.

80 Schapira DV, Kumar NB, Lyman GH, *et al.*: Abdominal obesity and breast cancer risk. *Ann Intern Med* 112: 182–186,1990.

81 Schapira DV, Kumar NB, Lyman GH, *et al.*: Obesity and body fat distribution and breast cancer prognosis. *Cancer* 67: 523–528,1991.

82 Sellers TA, Kushi LH, Potter JD, *et al.*: Effect of family history, body fat distribution, and reproductive factors on the risk of postmenopausal breast cancer. *N Engl J Med* 326: 1323–1329,1992.

83 Kumar NB, Lyman GH, Allen K, Cox CE, Schapira DV: Timing of weight gain and breast cancer risk. *Cancer* 76: 243–249,1995.

84 Stoll BA: Timing of weight gain in relation to breast cancer risk. *Ann Oncol* 6: 245–248,1995.

85 Frisch RE, Wyshak G, Albright NL, *et al.*: Lower lifetime occurrence of breast cancer and cancers of the reproductive system among former college athletes. *Am J Clin Nutr* 45: 328–335,1987.

86 Colditz G, Stampfer M, *et al.*: Prospective study of estrogen replacement therapy and the risk of breast cancer in postmenopausal women. *JAMA* 264: 2648–2652,1990.

11

Effects of exercise on the cardiovascular and osseous systems

PHILIP J BUCKENMEYER

INTRODUCTION

Women's health is increasingly becoming a priority for our growing and aging society. This is readily observed in funding programs for women's health, such as the NIH Women's Health Initiative. Until recent years, most research endeavors focused on men's health. Although men and women share similar health problems, gender differences should be recognized if clinicians are to treat patients appropriately. The basic physiology and hormonal milieu of men and women may contribute to or lessen the incidence of certain disease states. For example, the cardiovascular and osteoporotic risk for men and women may differ due to exogenous levels of estrogen and age. Several factors go into the process of keeping individuals healthy. Both pharmacologic and nonpharmacologic (for example, exercise and nutrition) approaches are being sought to optimize medical services.

It is also important to understand the health concerns of women as they exist within various socioeconomic communities. One study showed, through a postal questionnaire sent to 1649 women aged 20 to 60, that cancer merited highest priority for health care in Great Britain. Cardiovascular health and osteoporosis received lower priorities. However, lack of exercise was known as a risk factor for cardiovascular disease (CVD) and osteoporosis by 84.6% and 29% of the respondents, respectively. The promotion of hormone replacement therapy for prevention of CVD and osteoporosis was given a low priority, although its potential benefit to CVD was less well known by the respondents. This study clearly shows that it is important for clinicians to communicate with their patients and provide educational resources on women's health in their respective communities.

THE MORTALITY ISSUE OF WOMEN'S HEALTH AND EXERCISE

In the last 30 years, a large amount of epidemiological research has demonstrated a fairly consistent relationship between sedentary lifestyle and long-term health, particularly in men. More recently, these types of studies have begun to provide information dealing with a less active lifestyle and its long-term health effects on women. In a study by Blair and colleagues[2], low fitness level was found to be a statistically significant independent predictor of mortality in women. In fact, fit women with any combination of smoking, elevated blood pressure or elevated cholesterol level had lower death rates than less fit women with none of these characteristic risk factors for mortality. This finding in itself suggests that physicians should encourage sedentary women patients to become more physically active to reduce the potential risk of premature death.

DEFINING PHYSICAL ACTIVITY AND FITNESS

The biggest question that a clinician or any health professional may ask is: 'What constitutes being physically active?' From an epidemiological approach, a sedentary lifestyle has been defined as less than once per week of self-reported physical activity (aerobic in nature) or lack of sweat-related activity.[3] Physical fitness, on the other hand, has been defined simply as having the necessary attributes to perform physical activity.[4] Physical activity is any bodily movement produced by skeletal muscles that results in energy expenditure.[4] The definitions, although simple, take on very important meanings to one type of nonpharmacological approach to medicine – that is, achieving health through exercise, or a level of health-related fitness as it relates to disease prevention and health promotion. In order to guide us through this chapter, let us focus on health-related fitness as:

> A state characterized by (a) an ability to perform daily activities with vigor, and (b) a demonstration of traits and capacities that are associated with low risk of premature development of the hypokinetic diseases (that is those associated with physical inactivity).[5]

Although we have identified meanings for fitness related to health, it is sometimes more difficult to apply definitions to specific health-related ailments. When an attempt is made to utilize exercise, this decision will involve the specific components of exercise prescription, which include type, duration, intensity, frequency and progression of that activity required to elicit the healthful benefit desired. With these thoughts in mind, the focus of this chapter is to address the interaction between exercise and two integral systems of the body, cardiovascular and osseous, relative to women's health during the perimenopausal years.

1. THE CARDIOVASCULAR SYSTEM AND WOMEN'S HEALTH

The current status

Epidemiological literature has clearly shown that women tend to live longer than men. In the majority of industrialized countries, the largest gender differential for mortality is due to cardiovascular disease.[6] This is supported by the observation of higher death rates from arteriosclerotic and degenerative heart disease in men compared to women (see Figure

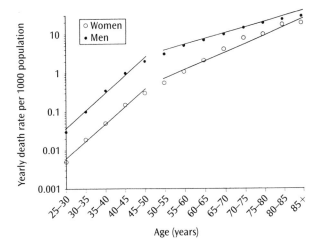

Figure 11.1 *Death rates from arteriosclerotic and degenerative heart disease in men compared to women relative to age. (Reproduced with permission from Heller RF, Jacobs HS. Coronary heart disease in relation to age, sex, and the menopause. BMJ 1978; 1: 472–474.)*

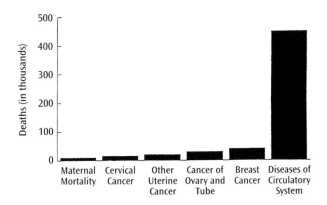

Figure 11.2 *Deaths among women in the United States via selected causes. (Reproduced with permission from Vital Statistics of the United States, 1981. Mortality. Part A. Ilyattsville, Maryland: National Center for Health Statistics, 1986.)*

11.1). Although this is true, death from cardiovascular disease still rates as an important health issue for women (Figure 11.2). Factors which place women at risk for CVD are elevated levels of body fat, higher blood pressure, higher plasma cholesterol levels, higher fibrinogen levels, and a higher incidence of diabetes compared to men.[6] Yet women tend to have favorable factors against cardiovascular risk, which include less upper body obesity, greater high-density lipoprotein (HDL), and lower triglyceride levels. It is believed that these more favorable factors can be explained, in part, by the hormone estrogen.[7]

As women enter into the perimenopausal years, the levels of endogenous estrogen begin to decline. Unfavorable lipid changes[8,9] (for example increase in LDL cholesterol – see Figure 11.3) and adverse shifts in the hemostatic factors fibrinogen and factor VII[10] have been shown to occur at the time of menopause. Due to the potential loss of estrogen's protective effect against cardiovascular disease, estrogen replacement therapy has been encouraged by many clinicians. Several investigations suggest positive benefits from estrogen

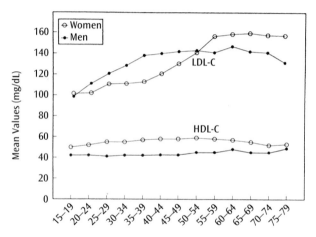

Figure 11.3 *Cholesterol lipoprotein fraction profile and age trends in men and women. (Reproduced with permission from Knopp RH, LaRosa JC, Burkman RT Jr. Contraception and dyslipidemia.* Am J Obstet Gynecol *1993; 168: 1994–2005.)*

replacement therapy, including significantly less heart disease and diabetes,[11] less athero-sclerosis[12] and an attenuated exercise-induced angina pectoris response.[13] Yet truly rando-mized placebo-controled clinical trials are still lacking.

The role of exercise

Large-scale prospective studies suggest a consistent reduction in heart disease with exercise in men and women.[14–17] Regular exercise has been shown to increase high-density lipo-protein (HDL) cholesterol and to decrease triglycerides. In addition, platelet adhesiveness is decreased and fibrinolysis is increased, which lessens the risk of atherosclerosis. It even lessens the adrenergic response to stress.[18] Despite these short-term benefits of regular exercise on cardiovascular risk factors, randomized clinical trials are lacking in finding the proof that exercise reduces cardiovascular risk. In fact, a cohort study from the Framing-ham group[19] showed no direct relationship between women who lived longer and decreased cardiovascular disease. The results of this investigation did, however, show that women who were more active had a higher survival rate (Figure 11.4).

Literature investigating the relationship between established cardiovascular risk factors and regular exercise in women is lacking, although a number of long-term investigations tend to support an inverse relationship. Blair and colleagues[2] have shown a protective effect of fitness for smokers, those with elevated cholesterol and unhealthy individuals in general. Total cholesterol, blood pressure and heart rate have been positively linked to the risk factor, total homocysteine, but all of these risk factors are inversely related to physical activity.[20] A Turkish study[21] suggests that hypertension and a lack of physical exercise constitute the most important risk factors, in addition to obesity. However, when account-ing for differences in body composition, that is, body mass index (BMI equals weight in kg divided by height in m[2]), the association between hypertension and physical activity appears to be attenuated.[22] A further evaluation of cardiovascular risk as it relates to physical activity in postmenopausal women showed that more fit individuals have a lessened cardiovascular risk.[23] In this study, all cardiovascular risk factors except for smoking showed more favorable associations with improved fitness in women compared to men.

Short-term studies also lend support to the positive effect of exercise on cardiovascular

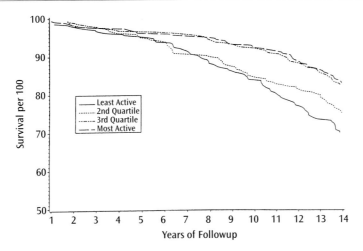

Figure 11.4 *Survival curves by physical activity quartiles in women during a 16-year follow-up. (Reproduced with permission from Sherman SE, D'Agostino RB, Cobb JL, Kannel WB. Physical activity and mortality in women in the Framingham Heart Study.* Am Heart J *1994; 128: 879–884.)*

risk factors. With five years of aerobic training, The Stanford Five-City Project resulted in increments of HDL cholesterol and decreased resting heart rate in women.[24] A 24-week diet and exercise study[25] was conducted on moderately obese postmenopausal women to determine if this group would receive similar benefits related to CVD risk factors that have been observed in premenopausal women. A significant amount of body weight was lost, but this risk factor was not accompanied by a reduction in other CVD risks. It is likely that the lack of endogenous estrogen may have accounted for this lack of change, or the exercise effort was not significant enough to elicit the desired changes.

Little information is known about habitual types of exercise training as it relates to CVD risk factors. A cross-sectional study of middle-aged women (in their forties) revealed that those who participated in resistance training (for example, weight lifting) elicited lower plasma cholesterol, LDL cholesterol and supine diastolic blood pressure compared to aerobically trained and untrained women.[26] Although this finding suggests that resistive training can be an effective means to achieve a beneficial cardiovascular risk profile, these results were primarily related to this group's lower amount of body fat. Another study of habitual exercisers showed that joggers had a more favorable risk profile compared to women who were regular participants in swimming, tennis, walking and calisthenics.[23] The importance of these studies is that certain types of physical activity may be more advantageous to cardiovascular health compared to others. Yet in order to answer this question, randomized longitudinal clinical trials need to be conducted.

The influence of exercise intensity on cardiovascular risk in postmenopausal women has not received much attention. However, a two-year study was conducted on 120 postmenopausal women to assess this exercise component.[27] Both high-intensity (three 40-minute endurance training sessions per week at 73% to 88% of peak treadmill heart rate) and low-intensity (five 30-minute endurance training sessions per week at 60% to 73% of peak treadmill heart rate) training were ineffective in changing HDL cholesterol after one year. However, at the end of two years of training, significant increases in HDL cholesterol levels and a lowered waist to hip ratio were observed. The increase in HDL cholesterol was more pronounced with low-intensity training. This study suggests that a longer time frame may be needed to elicit positive cardiovascular benefits from exercise in this age group compared to premenopausal women. In addition, frequency of participation appears to be an important factor in reducing cardiovascular risk. This notion is supported by an epidemiological study[22] which identified a high level of weekly exercise participation as greater than or equal to three times per week for periods of 20 minutes of exertion (described as shortness of breath, increase in pulse and perspiration).

The effectiveness of exercise in conjunction with hormone replacement therapy (HRT) in reducing cardiovascular disease risk is yet to be established. Premenopausal women, who already have a higher level of endogenous estrogens, appear to lack the more pronounced effect of an improved lipid profile that men have in response to regular exercise. Postmenopausal women without HRT have been shown to have a heightened response of HDL cholesterol to exercise.[28] Another study indicates a sluggish HDL response to moderate exercise.[29] This discrepancy appears to be the result of comparing a cross-sectional with a longitudinal intervention study.

Recommendations for women's cardiovascular health and exercise

Establishing exercise programs for perimenopausal women with the intention of reducing cardiovascular risk appears to have legitimate purpose. A realistic goal should be established that takes into account individual needs. These programs should include frequent sessions per week of aerobic exercise, as well as resistive exercise if desired by the patient. As noted in a combined statement by the Centers for Disease Control and Prevention and the American College of Sports Medicine, 30 minutes or more of moderate-intensity physical activity (equivalent to a brisk walk at 3 to 4 miles per hour) on most, preferably all, days of the week should be accumulated.[30] Prescribing exercise for women's health is an important challenge, especially when taking into account the hormonal factor difference between pre- and postmenopausal patients. All of the known facts regarding estrogen replacement therapy should be thoroughly discussed with the patient as we continue to explore its interaction with exercise.

II. THE OSSEOUS SYSTEM AND WOMEN'S HEALTH

The current status

Osteoporosis, along with cardiovascular disease and breast cancer, is one of the three most serious diseases facing women today. Some of the facts about this debilitating condition include: 1) approximately 21 million women in the U.S. are at high risk for osteoporosis; 2) nearly half of all women over the age of 50 will suffer a fracture associated with osteoporosis; 3) more than 1.5 million fractures occur per year, often resulting in painful and crippling hip fractures; 4) of those with resultant hip fractures, 20% die within a year and half of the survivors can never walk independently again; and 5) it incurs a nationwide annual medical cost of $10 billion.[31] In order to confront osteoporosis appropriately, we must first identify factors which have an influence on its risk. The determinants of osteoporosis risk for women in their peri- and postmenopausal years will depend upon several factors, which include peak bone mass achieved during the early years of life, genetic influences, hormonal status, dietary factors, exercise patterns, and sociological and environmental influences.[32] Figure 11.5 gives an indication of the general trend associated with bone status throughout a woman's lifetime.

Although this disease presents a significant medical problem to our society, proper intervention strategies involving diet, exercise and estrogen can make important

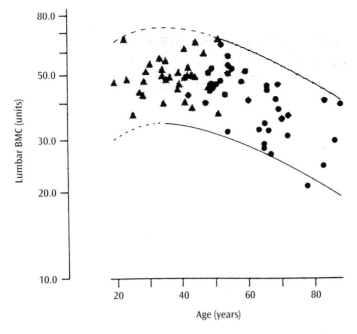

Figure 11.5 *General trend associated with bone status throughout a woman's lifetime. (Reproduced with permission from Krolner B, Pors Nielsen S. Bone mineral content of the lumbar spine in normal and osteoporotic women: cross-sectional and longitudinal studies.* Clin Sci. *1982; 62: 329–336.)*

contributions to its prevention and control. This section will focus primarily on the effect of exercise on osteoporotic risk, yet it should be clearly understood that exercise will be a more effective intervention if linked to individual nutritional and hormonal needs. This is particularly true in peri- and postmenopausal women. Women should be educated to and follow Recommended Dietary Allowance (RDA) recommendations for essential nutrients affecting bone health, which include calcium, phosphorus, and vitamins C and D.[33] The other factor which women, particularly in their menopausal years, should consider is the use of estrogen replacement therapy (ERT). It appears that this nonnutritional intervention can be effective in halting bone loss and reducing osteoporotic fractures,[34,35] however it does carry certain risks that should be discussed closely with the patient's physician. If ERT is not a viable option, other considerations may be possible, including newly developed drugs (calcitonin and Fosamax) and lifestyle changes such as cessation of smoking and participation in physical activities on a regular basis.

The role of exercise

Several exercise interventions have been carried out in an effort to determine if exercise is truly effective in promoting bone mass. In essence, there is general agreement that this can occur but is dependent upon the type, amount, duration and frequency of the exercise condition relative to different stages in a woman's life. Studies show that premenopausal women who exercise vigorously on a regular basis and have amenorrhea can lose bone mass. However, bone loss can be reversed or minimized with ERT in these women.[36,37] This finding suggests that exercise itself, in a state of estrogen deficiency, cannot prevent bone loss. Yet in a well-controlled investigation comparing the interactive effects of calcium, exercise and ERT on the prevention of bone loss, exercise alone did improve bone density in women with low bone mass.[38] However, the combination of the three independent variables resulted in optimal bone health.

Physical activity and the premenopausal years

In general, cross-sectional studies show that active women and athletes have a higher bone density than their sedentary peers,[39,40] although collegiate swimmers have been shown to have similar or lower vertebral bone mineral density compared to other athletes and control subjects.[41,42] This suggests that regularly performed weight-bearing activities may be advantageous to bone density gains. Studies of impact loading sports such as volleyball and gymnastics,[43] as well as squash, high-impact aerobics and speed skating,[44] support this notion. Vertebral and axial bone density gains in these studies range from 1% to 15% in young women athletes. Longitudinal studies, however, have not been very conclusive in identifying exercise as a significant promoter of bone mass gains. Mazess and Barden[45] did not find any relationship between moderate levels of aerobic activity and bone density change in lumbar spine, proximal femur or radius over the course of two years of training. Even more astounding, a 12-month study found no significant effect of Nautilus weight training on lumbar spine or os calcis bone mineral density.[46] Although an 83% increase in overall strength was observed, only a 0.8% increase was observed in vertebral bone and a 0.3% decrease occurred in os calcis bone density. It is unknown if changes occurred to axial bones (radius or femur); those bones supporting arm and leg muscular work. More longitudinal investigations need to be done in order to verify these findings.

Physical activity and the perimenopausal years

As with earlier years of life, active women during the perimenopausal period (around 35 to 50 years of age) tend to have higher bone mineral densities compared to their sedentary peers. In most cases, this is a result of a lifetime of regular physical activity which has led to a greater peak bone mass gain.[47] In a cross-sectional study,[48] runners were observed to have a higher radial bone mineral density (4.7%) compared to sedentary women, yet they had a lower os calcis density (by 6.8%) compared to their heavier inactive peers. One would expect to observe a greater bone density in the os calcis of the runners compared to the controls, yet this was not the case. This study suggests that body weight may actually have an overriding effect on change in bone density compared to that expected from the mechanical stress of exercise. Another study[49] has shown a significant relationship between total body calcium and lumbar bone density with physical activity, although the correlations were quite low. These low correlations were linked to the low physical activity levels recorded by the investigators. Longitudinal studies are lacking in this age group, although one study utilized a nine-month structured weight training program to investigate bone response.[50] Surprisingly, decreases in lumbar spine (by 4%) and femoral neck (by 1%) bone densities were observed, even though strength increased by 57%. It is plausible that the strength training period was not long enough or intensive enough to elicit bone density gains. An unaccounted factor may be a decrement in estrogen status, which the researchers did not address.

Physical activity and the postmenopausal years

Increased interest in the potential effectiveness of ERT in slowing down the osteoporotic condition has generated a number of investigations. Some of these studies have focused on whether exercise alone can be effective or whether it is more effective in conjunction with ERT. Most cross-sectional studies in this age group are equivocal. In studies involving Masters runners, 35%[51] and 9.2%[52] gains in lumbar bone density have been observed in active exercisers compared to age-matched controls. These results may reflect increases in bone mass achieved through habitual physical activity since earlier years of life. Supportive of these findings, more fit women have been shown to have an 18% higher calcium bone index (via neutron activation) at the trunk and proximal femur[53] and an 18% greater cortical width of the second metacarpal.[54] Contrary to these findings, another study involving postmenopausal runners showed no difference in lumbar spine or radial bone mineral density when compared to a sedentary age-matched control group.[55] Additionally, when the older runners were compared to a group of younger runners, lumbar spine and radial bone densities were 39% and 16% lower in the postmenopausal group (Table 11.1). This study suggests that without estrogen, exercise is not effective in preventing bone loss. Yet, a recent epidemiological survey suggests the beneficial influence of exercise on bone mineral density and its ability for preventing bone loss.[56]

Strength training has been perceived as a means to improve bone health, particularly in younger athletes. The relationship of muscular strength to bone mineral density in post-menopausal women has met with mixed results. Some investigations report a significant correlation[57,58] while another study[59] casts doubt in a muscular strength-bone density connection. Differences in measurement techniques, selection bias and identification of strength training methodologies need to be controlled in order clearly to determine if weight training is effective in protecting postmenopausal women from bone loss.

The addition of hormone replacement therapy to the exercise variable has shown benefits in postmenopausal women.[60,61] In one study,[61] nonestrogen-repleted swimmers had only a 0.9% greater vertebral bone density compared to nonexercisers; however, with estrogen therapy, swimmers had a 4% advantage over nonswimmers. An 11% difference in lumbar spine density was noted between estrogen-repleted versus estrogen-deficient swimmers. As noted with Master's runners, postmenopausal swimmers without ERT had significantly lower vertebral bone density compared to premenopausal swimmers. Thus, this study suggests that habitual exercise (swimming) does not prevent bone loss with age, but it does appear to have an additive effect with ERT. ERT plus a circuit weight training program also seems to provide a boost in bone density in postmenopausal women.[62] An 8.4% increment in lumbar spine bone density was observed in this study.

Table 11.1 *Comparison of older versus younger women runners relative to lumbar spine and radial bone densities. (Reproduced with permission from Kirk S, Sharp CF, Elbaum N, Endres DB, Simons SM, Mohler JG, Rude RK. Effect of long-distance running on bone mass in women.* J Bone Miner Res *1989; 4: 515–522.)*

Age (years)	VBD (mg/cm^3)^a	CBD (gm/cm^2)	VO$_{2max}$ (ml/kg per minute)
25–35			
Runners	183 ± 7^b	0.738 ± 0.01	48 ± 1^c
Sedentary	163 ± 8	0.732 ± 0.01	32 ± 2
55–65			
Runners	112 ± 5	0.617 ± 0.03	37 ± 2^c
Sedentary	111 ± 5	0.665 ± 0.04	24 ± 2

^{a} Values are means ± SEM.
^{b} $t = 1.99$, $p = 0.0778$ compared with sedentary controls.
^{c} Significantly different from sedentary, $p < 0.01$.

These types of exercise programs deserve further study in an effort to verify the additive effect of hormone replacement therapy with exercise.

Preliminary longitudinal studies tended to support the contention that exercise programs do not prevent bone loss in postmenopausal women.[63,64] However, the addition of calcium and vitamin D3 supplements to exercise has proven effective in improving vertebral and femoral bone mineral density[64,65] and in slowing the rate of radial bone loss.[38] Other longitudinal studies refute the notion that exercise is not effective, in and of itself, in promoting positive bone health. In a two-year, twice-weekly, aerobic, weight-bearing exercise program, a 9.6% increase in trochanteric bone density was observed in post-menopausal women compared to a 4.4% loss in an age-matched nonexercising control group.[66] Positive outcomes of bone health have also been cited from less notable types of regular exercise programs for postmenopausal women, such as aerobics,[67] calisthenics,[68] stair climbing,[69] weight lifting[67,70] and dancing.[71]

Recommendations for women's osseous health and exercise

Like cardiovascular health, osseous health is a long-term process beginning early in a woman's life. The keys to optimal bone health are dependent upon the successful interaction between diet, exercise and estrogen. Relative to the exercise component, peri- and postmenopausal women should consider participating in both 'weight bearing' aerobic exercise as well as 'resistive' weight training. Aerobic exercise (for example, brisk walking) should be performed for 30 minutes or more for most days during the week.[30] Based on recommendations from the American College of Sports Medicine,[72] resistive training sessions of 20 to 30 minutes' duration should be performed at least twice per week, with at least 48 hours of rest between sessions. Sessions longer than 60 minutes may affect long-term adherence to this type of training. It is recommended that one set of eight to 10 exercises involving the major muscle groups (that is, quadriceps, hamstrings, pectorals, latissimus dorsi, deltoids, abdominals, gluteals) be performed. Upper and lower body exercises should be alternated to allow short-term recovery of exercised muscles. Each exercise within the set should be performed eight to 12 times (repetitions) at an exertion level that feels 'somewhat hard'. Simple resistance exercises can utilize body weight, hand-held weights, and thera-bands as effective starting weight resistance devices. In prescribing exercise, individuals needs should be taken into account and should be discussed closely with patients' physician and supportive health profesionals. This is also true when considering calcium intake and estrogen replacement therapy as additive factors to exercise, as these factors may provide the most advantageous means of approaching optimal bone health.

REFERENCES

1 Griffiths F: Women's health concerns. Is the promotion of hormone replacement therapy for prevention important to women? *Fam Pract* 12(1): 54–59,1995.
2 Blair SN, Kampert JB, Kohl HW 3rd, Barlow CE, Macera CA, Paffenbarger RS Jr, Gibbons LW: Influences of cardiorespiratory fitness and other precursors on cardiovascular disease and all-cause mortality in men and women. *JAMA* 276(3): 205–210,1996.
3 Eaton CB, Lapane KL, Garber CA, Assaf AR, Lasater TM, Carleton RA: Sedentary lifestyle and risk of coronary heart disease in women. *Med Sci Sports Exerc* 27(11): 1535–1539,1995.
4 Casperson CJ, Powell KE, Christenson GM: Physical activity, exercise and physical fitness: Definitions and distinctions for health-related research. *Public Health Reports* 100: 126–131,1985.

5 Pate RR: The evolving definition of physical fitness. *Quest* 40: 174–179,1988.

6 Barrett-Connor E: Heart disease in women. *Fertil Steril* 62(2): 127S–132S,1994.

7 Wild RA, Taylor EL, Knehans A: The gynecologist and cardiovascular disease: A window of opportunity for prevention. *J Soc Gynecol Invest* 1: 103–117,1994.

8 Kannel WB: Nutrition and the occurrence and prevention of cardiovascular disease in the elderly. *Nutr Rev* 46: 68–78,1988.

9 Matthews KA, Meilahn E, Kuller LH, Kelsey SF, Caggiula AW, Wing RR: Menopause and risk factors for coronary heart disease. *N Engl J Med* 321: 641–646,1989.

10 Meilahn EN, Kuller LH, Matthews KA, Kiss JE: Hemostatic factors according to menopausal status and use of hormone replacement therapy. *Ann Epidemiol* 2: 445–455,1992.

11 Hammond CV, Jelovsek FR, Lee KL, Creasman WT, Parker RT: Effects of long-term estrogen replacement therapy, I: metabolic effects. *AM J Obstet Gynecol* 133: 525–536,1979.

12 Stampfer MJ, Colditz GA: Estrogen replacement therapy and coronary disease: A quantitative assessment of the epidemiological evidence. *Prev Med* 20: 47–63,1991.

13 Rosano GM, Sarrell PM, Poole-Wilson PA, Collins P: Beneficial effects of estrogen on exercise-induced myocardial ischemia on women with coronary artery disease. *Lancet* 342: 133–136,1993.

14 Slattery ML, Jacobs DR Jr, Nichaman MZ: Leisure time physical activity and coronary heart disease death: the US railroad study. *Circulation* 79: 304–311,1989.

15 Leon AS, Connet J, Jacobs DR, Raumaraa R: Leisure-time physical activity levels and risk of coronary heart disease and death: The multiple risk factor intervention trial. *JAMA* 258: 2388–2395,1987.

16 Kannel WB, Sorlie P: Some health benefits of physical activity: The Framingham Study. *Arch Intern Med* 139: 857–861,1979.

17 Paffenbarger RS Jr, Hyde RT, Wing AL, Hsieh C–c: Physical activity, all-cause mortality, and longevity of college alumni. *N Engl J Med* 314: 605–613,1986.

18 Cooksey JD, Reilly P, Brown S, Bomze H, Cryer PE: Exercise training and plasma catecholamines in patients with ischemic heart disease. *Am J Cardiol* 42: 372–376,1978.

19 Sherman SE, D'Agostino RB, Cobb JL, Kannel WB: Physical activity and mortality in women in the Framingham Heart Study. *Am Heart J* 128: 879–884,1994.

20 Nygard O, Vollset SE, Refsum H, Stensvold I, Tverdal A, Nordrehaug JE, Ueland M, Kvale G: Total plasma homocysteine and cardiovascular risk profile. The Hordaland Homocysteine Study. *JAMA* 274 (19): 1526–1533,1995.

21 Onat A, Senocak MS: Relative risk of factors for coronary heart disease in population with low cholesterol levels. *Int J Cardiol* 43 (1): 51–60,1994.

22 Hong Y, Bots ML, Pan X, Wang H, Jing H, Hofman A, Chen H: Physical activity and cardiovascular risk factors in rural Shanghai, China. *Int J Epidemiol* 23 (6): 1154–1158,1994.

23 Bovens AM, Van Baak MA, Vrencken JG, Wijnen JA, Saris WH, Verstappen FT: Physical activity, fitness, and selected risk factors for CHD in active men and women. *Med Sci Sports Exerc* 25(5): 572–576,1993.

24 Young DR, Haskell WL, Jatulis DE, Fortmann SP: Associations between changes in physical activity and risk factors for coronary heart disease in a community-based sample of men and women: The Stanford Five-City Project. *Am J Epidemiol* 138 (4): 205–216,1993.

25 Fox AA, Thompson JL, Butterfield GE, Gylfadottir U, Moynihan S, Spiller G: Effects of diet and exercise on common cardiovascular disease risk factors in moderately obese older women. *Am J Clin Nutr* 63 (2): 225–233,1996.

26 Toth MJ, Poehlman ET: Resting metabolic rate and cardiovascular disease risk in resistance- and aerobic-training middle-aged women. *Int J Obes relat Metab Disord* 19 (10): 691–698,1995.

27 King AC, Haskell WL, Young DR, Oka RK, Stefanick ML: Long-term effects of varying intensities and formats of physical activity on participation rates, fitness, and lipoproteins in men and women aged 50–65 years. *Circulation* 91 (10): 2596–2604,1995.

28 Hartung GH, Moore CE, Mitchell R, Kappus CM: Relationship of menopausal status and exercise level to HDL cholesterol in women. *Exp Aging Res* 10: 13–18,1984.

29 Cauley JA, Kriska AM, LaPorta RE, Sandler RB, Pambianco G: A two-year randomized exercise trial in older women: Effects on HDL-cholesterol. *Atheroslerosis* 66: 247–258,1987.

30 Pate RR, Pratt M, Blair SN, *et al.*: Physical Activity and Public Health: A recommendation from the Centers for Disease Control and Prevention and the American College of Sports Medicine. *JAMA* 273: 402–407,1995.

31 McBean LD, Forgac T, Finn SC: Osteoporosis: Visions for care and prevention – a conference report. *J Am Diet Assoc* 94: 668–671,1994.

32 Lappe JM: Bone fragility: Assessment of risk and strategies for prevention. *J Obset Gynecol Neonat Nurs* 23 (3): 260–268,1994.

33 Heaney RP: Nutritional factors in osteoporosis. *Ann Rev Nutr* 13: 287–316,1993.

34 Ettinger B, Genant HK, Cann CE: Postmenopausal bone loss is prevented by treatment with low-dosage estrogen with calcium. *Ann Intern Med* 106: 40–45,1987.

35 Ravnikar V: Hormonal management of osteoporosis. *Clin Obstet Gynecol* 35: 913–922,1992.

36 Drinkwater BL, Nilson K, Chestnut CH III, Bremner J, Shainholtz S, Southworth MB: Bone mineral content of amenorrheic and eumenorrheic athletes. *N Engl J Med* 311: 277–281,1984.

37 Drinkwater BL, Nilson K, Ott S, Chestnut CH III: Bone mineral density after resumption of menses in amenorrheic women. *JAMA* 256: 380–382,1986.

38 Prince R, Smith M, Dick IM, Price RI, Webb PG, Henderson K, Harris M: Prevention of osteoporosis: A comparative study of exercise, calcium supplementation, and hormone-replacement therapy. *N Engl J Med* 325: 1189–1195,1991.

39 Heinrich CH, Going SB, Parmenter RW, Perry CD, Boyden TW, Lohman TG: Bone mineral content of cyclically menstruating female resistant and endurance trained athletes. *Med Sci Sports Exerc* 22: 558–563,1990.

40 Jacobsen PC, Beaver W, Grubb SA, Taft TN, Talmage RV: Bone density in women: College athletes and older athletic women. *J Orthop Res* 2: 328–332,1984.

41 Rourke KM, Bowering J, Turkki P, Buckenmeyer PJ, Thomas FD, Keller BA, Sforzo BA: Bone mineral density in weight-bearing and overweight-bearing female athletes. *Paediatric Exercise* 10: 28–37,1998.

42 Risser WL, Lee EJ, LeBlanc A, Poindexter HB, Risser JMH, Schneider V: Bone density in eumenorrheic female college athletes. *Med Sci Sports Exerc* 22: 570–574,1990.

43 Fehling PC, Alekel L, Clasey J, Rector A, Stillman RJ: A comparison of bone mineral densities among female athletes in impact loading and active loading sports. *Bone* 17: 205–210,1995.

44 Heinonen A, Oja P, Kannus P, Sievanen H, Haapasalo H, Manttari A, Vuori I: Bone mineral density in female athletes representing sports with different loading characteristics of the skeleton. *Bone* 17: 197–203,1995.

45 Mazess RB, Barden HS: Bone density in premenopausal women: Effect of age, dietary intake, physical activity, smoking, and birth-control pills. *Am J Clin Nutr* 53: 132–142,1991.

46 Gleeson PB, Portas EJ, LeBlanc A, Schneider VS, Evans HJ: Effects of weight lifting on bone mineral density in premenopausal women. *J Bone Miner Res* 5: 153–158,1990.

47 Stevenson JC, Lees B, Devenport M, Cust MP, Ganger KF: Determinants of bone density in normal women: risk factors for future osteoporosis? *Br Med J* 298: 924–928,1989.

48 Brewer V, Meyer BM, Keele MS, Upton SJ, Hagan RD: Role of exercise in prevention of involutional bone loss. *Med Sci Sports Exerc* 15: 445–449,1983.

49 Aloia JF, Vaswani AN, Yeh J, Cohn SH: Premenopausal bone mass is related to physical activity. *Arch Intern Med* 148: 121–123,1988.

50 Rockwell JC, Sorensen AM, Bakier S, Lehey D, Stock JL, Michaels J, Baran DT: Weight training decreases vertebral bone density in premenopausal women: A prospective study. *J Clin Endocrinol Metab.* 71: 988–993,1990.

51 Lane NE, Bloch DA, Jones HH, Marshall WH, Wood PD, Fries JF: Long-distance running, bone density, and osteoarthritis. *JAMA* 255: 1147–1151,1986.

52 Michel BA, Bloch DA, Fries JF: Weight–bearing exercise, overexercise, and lumbar bone density over age 50 years. *Arch Intern Med* 149: 2325–2329,1989.

53 Chow RK, Harrison JE, Brown CF, Hajek V: Physical fitness effect on bone mass in postmenopausal women. *Arch Phys Med Rehabil 67: 231–234,1986.*

54 Oyster N, Morton M, Linnell S: Physical activity and osteoporosis in postmenopausal women. *Med Sci Sports Exerc* 16: 44–50,1984.

55 Kirk S, Sharp CF, Elbaum N, Endres DB, Simons SM, Mohler JG, Rude RK: Effect of long-distance running on bone mass in women. *J Bone Miner Res* 4: 515–522,1989.

56 Kane K: Relationship between exercise and bone mineral density among over 5000 women aged 40 years and above. *J Epidemiol* 8: 28–32,1998.

57 Pocock NA, Eisman J, Gwinn T, Sambrook P, Kelly P, Freund J, Yeates M: Muscle strength, physical fitness, and weight but not age predict femoral neck bone mass. *J Bone Miner* 4: 441–448,1989.

58 Sinaki M, Offord KP: Physical activity in postmenopausal women: Effect on back muscle strength and bone mineral density of the spine. *Arch Phys Med Rehabil* 69: 277–280,1988.

59 Bevier WC, Wiswell RA, Pyka G, Kozak KC, Newhall KM, Marcus R: Relationship of body composition, muscle strength, and aerobic capacity to bone mineral density in older men and women. *J Bone Miner Res* 4: 421–432,1989.

60 Kohrt WM, Ehsani AA, Birge SJ Jr: HRT preserves increases in bone mineral density and reductions in body fat after supervised exercise program. *J Appl Physiol* 84: 1506–1512,1998.

61 Orwell ES, Ferar J, Oviatt SK, McClung MR, Huntingdon K: The relationship of swimming exercise to bone mass in men and women. *Arch Intern Med* 149: 2197–2200,1989.

62 Notelovitz M, Martin D, Tesar R, McKenzie L, Fields C: Estrogen therapy and variable resistance weight training increases bone mineral in surgically menopausal women. *J Bone Miner Res* 6: 583–590,1991.

63 Cavanaugh DJ, Cann CE: Brisk walking does not stop bone loss in postmenopausal women. *Bone* 9: 201–204,1988.

64 Nelson ME, Fisher EC, Dilmanian FA, Dallal GE, Evans WJ: A 1-y walking program and increased calcium in postmenopausal women: Effects on bone. *AM J Clin Nutr* 53: 1304–1311,1991.

65 Iwamoto J, Takeda T, Otani T, Yabe Y: Effect of increased physical activity on bone mineral density in postmenopausal osteoporotic women. *Koio J Med* 47: 157–161,1998.

66 Caplan GA, Ward JA, Lord SR: The benefits of exercise in postmenopausal women. *Aust J Public Health* 17 (1): 23–26,1993.

67 Chow RK, Harrison JE, Notarius C: Effect of two randomised exercise programmes on bone mass of healthy postmenopausal women. *Br Med J* 295: 1441–1444,1987.

68 Krolner B, Toft B, Nielsen SP, Tondevold E: Physical exercise as prophylaxis against involutional vertebral bone loss: A controlled trial. *Clin Sci* 64: 541–546,1983.

69 Dalsky G, Stocke KS, Eshani AA, Slatopolsky E, Lee WC, Birge SJ: Weight-bearing exercise training and lumbar bone mineral content in postmenopausal women. *Ann Intern Med* 1908: 824–828,1988.

70 Ayalon J, Simkin A, Leichter I, Raifmann S: Dynamic bone loading exercises for postmenopausal women: Effect on the density of the distal radius. *Arch Phys Med Rehabil* 68: 280–283,1987.

71 Peterson SE, Peterson MD, Raymond G, Gilligan C, Checovich MM, Smith EL: Muscular strength and bone density with weight training in middle-aged women. *Med Sci Sports Exerc* 23: 499–504,1991.

72 American College of Sports Medicine: *Guidelines for Exercise Testing and Prescription.* fifth ed. Media, PA: Williams and Wilkins, 1995.

12

Hormone replacement therapy: an overview

RAJA W ABDUL-KARIM, SAMUEL S BADALIAN AND

SHYLAJA MAINI

INTRODUCTION

A chapter on hormone replacement therapy cannot be all-encompassing, for it embodies a wide range of interrelated subjects, each worthy of a disquisition on its own. Consequently and in good faith, an element of selection in both the theme and depth of discussion must enter the picture. It is our intent to offer an explication of the principles governing hormone replacement therapy and its ramifications.

The phrase 'hormone replacement therapy' is generic. Nonetheless, it has become synonymous with the regimen of medications given to women specifically because of waning estrogen production consequent to ovarian extirpation or aging. The phrase is a misnomer, for none of the currently used regimens mimic normal ovarian function. The cornerstone of hormone replacement therapy (HRT) is estrogen. The function of progestins is chiefly to protect the endomentrium from the effects of chronic exposure to estrogens, and the routine use of androgens is still in debate.

The 'standard' dose of estrogen in prevailing HRT regimens is based primarily on the lowest dosage that serves as an adequate prophylaxis against osteoporosis. This point is important, for the estrogen dose addresses directly only one consequence of menopause (namely, accelerated bone loss), and is not necessarily the optimate dosage for managing other sequelae of the menopause (for example, urogenital atrophy). The situation becomes even more cloudy when other potential effects of estrogens are considered which do not constitute an approved indication for estrogen use. Presently, there is compelling evidence supporting a beneficial cardiovascular effect for estrogens. On less firm ground, but consistent with emerging data, are other equally exciting possible advantages to estrogen use after menopause (for example, improving memory, prevention and/or amelioration of Alzheimer's disease, maintaining skin and collagen integrity and a female pattern of fat distribution, and improving the digestion and absorption of nutrients). The optimal dosage of estrogen for any of these potential benefits has not been determined.

The preceding discussion attempts to place 'hormone replacement therapy' in proper perspective. We favor the more discursive 'estrogen replacement therapy' (ERT). However, HRT has become firmly entrenched in both medical and nonmedical parlance; hence HRT and ERT will be used interchangeably in this chapter.

ESTROGENS

Estrogens are not a homogenous group. They may be steroidal or nonsteroidal compounds, and may differ in their origin (plant, animal or synthetic), relative potency, and side effects. This aspect is worth remembering, since some of the concerns regarding HRT have been unfairly extrapolated from differing estrogen/progestin regimens. The ideal estrogen to administer in ERT would be that selected for a specific effect(s) with no untoward side effects. Regrettably, such an estrogen does not exist.

From a clinical point of view, estrogens may be divided into three categories: 1) natural (for example, estradiol, estone, estriol, equilin, equilenin); 2) synthetic analogues of natural estrogens (for example, ethinyl estradiol, methyl ethinyl estradiol); 3) synthetic (for example, diethylstilbestrol, hexestrol). With rare exceptions, only the natural estrogens should be used in HRT.

Mechanisms of action

The mechanism(s) by which estrogens exert their effects at the cellular level has not been elucidated completely for all of the compounds, but has been most extensively studied for the steroidal hormones. The latter were believed to exert their effects by binding to intracellular receptors, whereas polypeptide hormones bind to receptors located in the cell membrane, generating a second messenger such as cyclic AMP. It is now clear that this distinction between the mechanisms of action of steroid and peptide hormones is not absolute and that steroidal estrogens exert their function by more than one mechanism.

1 **Steroid receptor-gene transcription interaction.** This is probably the most prevalent mechanism. In simplified form, it involves the following steps: 1) the passage of the estrogen through the cell membrane and 2) binding to its receptor protein forming a steroid receptor complex that 3) enter the nucleus and binds to chromatin acceptors, 4) initiating the transcription of specific messenger RNA. Recently, a second estrogen receptor has been identified, as well as an estrogen receptor regulatory pathway not mediated by the estrogen response element[1,2]
2 **Steroid membrane receptor interaction.** Estrogen receptor binding sites that do not translocate into the nucleus have been identified on the cell membrane. This may explain responses to estrogens occurring too rapidly to be explained by a mechanism

involving gene transcription. Such effects may be consequent to the steroid binding to receptors in plasma, lysomal or mitochondrial membranes.[3]

3 **Stimulation of cAMP.** Estradiol, in physiologic concentrations, increases adenylate cyclase activity and stimulates cAMP. A dose-response relationship is present. This effect is not dependent on antecedent RNA or protein synthesis. The increase in adenylate cyclase activity in response to estrogen suggests a possible action on the cell membrane. Estrogens vary in their potency to stimulate cyclic AMP[4] estradiol 17β > diethylstilbestrol > 2-OH estrone > estradiol 17α). The intracellular increase in cAMP may modulate cAMP-influenced activities, including the expression of genes.

Thus it is apparent that the aftermaths of estrogens are mediated via more than one mechanism. Experimentally, estrogen influences have been described in all body systems. Accordingly, when estrogen deficiency occurs in women, the consequences are not limited to the reproductive tract or secondary sexual characteristics. Although the indications for estrogen replacement therapy are limited to: 1) hot flushes, 2) vulvar, vaginal, urethral atrophy, 3) prevention and treatment of osteoporosis, 4) hypoestrogenism due to gonadectomy or ovarian failure, it is anticipated that the indications for estrogens will expand in the not-too-distant future.

Relative potency

The potency of an estrogen is related to how long the ER complex resides in the nucleus. Potency, however, is relative, since it depends on the target and the estrogen and, under ideal circumstances, should direct the choice of the estrogen for the appropriate target.

There is not a plethora of studies comparing the relative potency of estrogens. Hammond and Maxon[5] summarized data on the relative potency of estradiol, estrone, ethinyl estradiol and mestranol on vaginal cornification and gonadotropin, implantation and ovulation suppression. Assigning estradiol a relative strength of 100 per cent for each of these endpoints, the relative strength of estrone was: 30, 30, 70, 150; of estriol: 3, 10, 12, 15; of ethinyl estradiol: 150, 300, 70, 170; and of mestranol: 10, 100, 20, 85, respectively.

In the same year, Mashchak and colleagues[6] reported on the relative potency of various estrogens on serum FSH, corticosteroid binding globulin (CBG), sex hormone binding globulin (SHBG) and angiotensinogen in healthy, postmenopausal women. Compared to piperazine estrone sulfate, micronized estradiol was equally potent with respect to SHBG, less potent with respect to angiotensinogen, and nearly twice as effective with respect to CBG. DES was more potent in all parameters, and ethinyl estradiol had the highest relative potency.

Relative potency is demonstrable in other systems. For example, equilin (a component of conjugated equine estrogens) has greater neurotrophic effects than 17β estradiol on neurons from several regions of the cerebral cortex, and is a more potent antioxidant than either 17β estradiol or estrone.[7,8]

PROGESTINS

Although progestins may have a favorable effect on bone density and can decrease the frequency and intensity of hot flushes, the principle use of progestins as part of HRT is to protect the endometrium from the effects of unopposed estrogen. Progestins may induce various side effects, such as abdominal bloating, headaches, irritability, a feeling of depression, lethargy, bloating and breast tenderness. In addition, the withdrawal bleeding associated with the cyclic use of progestins may be bothersome to some women. Such side effects may be sufficiently troublesome to induce their sufferers to discontinue the hormonal regimen. Sometimes, reduction in the progestin dosage or changing the progestin used for another, eliminates the undesirable symptoms or ameliorates them to the degree of tolerability. In any case, the progestin used must fulfil its primary role, namely, protecting the endometrium. In the absence of the uterus, there is no clear, established benefit to the use of progestins. Where estrogens may be contraindicated, progestins can ameliorate hot flushes. Although of no *proven* benefit, the use of progestins may be prudent in women with a recent history of endometriosis or a history of endometroid ovarian cancer or endometrial cancer, should hormone replacement therapy be considered in these patients. The final word has not been written on this subject, and a clear discourse of pros and cons should occur between patient and physician.

Types of progestins

From a clinical perspective, progestins used in HRT regimens may be divided into three categories: 1) progesterone, 2) 19-norprogestins (for example, norgestrel or norethindrone), 3) C-21 progestins (for example, medroxyprogesterone acetate, megestrol acetate).

PROGESTERONE

Of the progestational agents, progesterone has the least adverse effect on lipoproteins. In the dosages employed, no adrogenicity or adverse effect on lipoproteins is demonstrable. The availability of progesterone in the micronized form has increased its absorption when given orally, although marked differences can occur among subjects and in a given individual. Doses in the range of 200 to 400 mg daily (orally) for 14 days, protect the endometrium against the effects of unopposed estrogen. Our limited experience with oral progesterone in HRT has shown this to be a good alternative to other more established progestational agents. We have frequently used the compound via the vaginal route in lower dosage and have been very satisfied with the results.

19-NORPROGESTINS

Primarily the progestin component in oral contraceptives, 19-norprogestins are more androgenic than either of the other two categories and have an adverse effect on lipoproteins. More frequently used in Europe than the United States in estrogen replacement regimes, 19-norprogestins are more reliably absorbed and, hence, exhibit a more consistent effect than either progesterone or medoxyprogesterone acetate. However, in view of their adverse effects on lipoproteins and their androgenicity, we recommend that these compounds be reserved for those situations where other progestational agents are not well tolerated. A daily dose of 0.35 mg of norethindrone or 0.075 mg of levonorgestrel administered alongside the estrogen is probably sufficient to protect the endometrium. Higher dosages are necessary in cyclic regimens.

C-21 PROGESTINS

Medroxyprogesterone acetate is the most commonly used and extensively studied progestin in hormone replacement therapy. Medroxyprogesterone acetate is rapidly absorbed with a half-life of approximately eight hours. In continuous regimens, 2.5 mg daily is usually sufficient; whereas in cyclic regimens, a minimum of 5 mg should be used for 12 and, preferably, 14 days each cycle. Differences in patient response are not infrequent, and the dosage may have to be adjusted accordingly (for example, 5 mg in the continuous and 10 mg for the cyclic regimens).

WHEN TO BEGIN HRT

Estrogen replacement therapy should begin with the diagnosis of menopause. The majority of menopaused women will respond to the usual regimens (see below); the remainder will continue to experience vasomotor symptoms. The addition of 0.3 mg of conjugated equine estrogens or 0.5 mg of 17β estradiol orally will control the symptoms in the majority of women. Young women experiencing surgical menopause require a higher dosage of estrogen than those with 'natural' menopause. For the former, the recommended daily dose is 1.25 mg of conjugated equine estrogens or 2 mg of 17β estradiol, or their equivalents, given orally; or 0.1 mg per 24 hours of 17β estradiol transdermally.

Along with the uterus, the vagina, vulva, urethra and trigone of the bladder undergo atrophy after menopause. Atrophy may actually begin prior to cessation of menses, with some women experiencing mild, often intermittent, dyspareunia. The dyspareunia, not uncommonly, is aggravated after menopause, and the atrophy of the urethral and bladder mucosa increases the risk of urinary tract infections and stress incontinence. Treatment for the consequences of urogenital atrophy often necessitates a higher amount of estrogen than usually prescribed in the 'classic' hormone replacement therapy regimens and the vaginal route is preferable because of local effect. Although primarily guided by the response of the patient, we have found that maintaining a blood level of estradiol somewhere between 80 and 115 picograms per milliliter is often necessary to achieve a desired response. For vulvo-vaginal atrophy, local estrogen application offers a better alternative to an incremental increase in systemically administered estrogens. Estriol cream is reportedly effective.

Increasing the dose of estrogen merits thoughtful attention. Are the risks of breast and endometrial cancer increased? Current knowledge does not provide a satisfactory answer. It should be noted that estrogens administered vaginally raise similar concerns, since they are absorbed quite efficiently from the vagina. We recommend increasing the dose of progestin, although this poses its own risk of undesirable side effects. Thus, in the absence of a compass to steer the physician, a constant adjustment of the therapeutic course is necessary, where risks are weighed against benefits.

Estrogen augmentation is often necessary prior to menopause. The waning hormonal functions of the ovary, characterized by menstrual irregularities, elevated FSH, and normal LH levels during the perimenopausal years, can lead to vasomotor instability of sufficient annoyance to warrant therapy. Our experience indicates that a daily oral dose of 0.3 mg of conjugated equine estrogens or 0.5 mg of 17β estradiol offers relief in the majority of instances and has no apparent shortcomings.

ESTROGEN REPLACEMENT THERAPY

Background

Estrogen replacement regimens are primarily the outgrowth of studies determining the minimum dosage of estrogen necessary for the prevention (or treatment) of postmenopausal osteoporosis. The dose of the accompanying progestin is based on the lowest dosage that effectively prevents endometrial hyperplasia. The stage for such studies may have been set by Albright and coworkers[9,10], who observed an association between osteoporosis and menopause. The ensuing years established the importance of estrogen in both the pre- and postnatal development of bone.[11–13]

If it seems that inordinate import is being granted to the relationship between estrogens and bone formation, this is intentional since, essential to the proper treatment of per- and postmenopausal women is an understanding of the diversity of the studies that are the foundation for HRT regimens. Whether the regimens used for osseous health are also optimal for cardiovascular and other systems' health remains to be seen. It is anticipated that this area will receive focused attention comparable to that given to the skeletal system.

One of the earliest attempts to establish the minimum effective dose of estrogen in the prevention of osteoporosis was carried out by Lindsay and coworkers in 1984.[14] The study included women who had had bilateral oophorectomy (62%) or had achieved natural menopause. The mean time lapsed since the LMP was 20 months, plus or minus 2.59 months. The subjects were divided into a control and four treatment groups. At the end of two years, bone density measurements by single photon absorptiometry was performed on the midpoint of the third right metacarpal bone. Subjects receiving the 0.15 mg or the 0.3 mg dose of the estrogens had a significant decrease in bone mineral density; whereas the bone mineral density in those receiving either the 0.625 mg or the 1.25 mg dose showed no change. Thus the minimum effective dose of conjugated equine estrogens that prevented bone loss was 0.625 mg per day (at least for the metacarpal bone, and over a two-year period).

Lindsay's findings are in general agreement with those of Genant and coworkers,[15] who studied women within two months of undergoing bilateral oophorectomy (mean age 42 years). Conjugated equine estrogens were given daily in doses of either 0.15, 0.3, 0.45, or 0.6 mg per day. Bone mineral density was measured in the lumbar spine (vertebrae 1 and 2), as well as in the second metacarpal bone and the distal end of the radial disphyses. At the end of two years, all women in the placebo group as well as those receiving less than 0.6 mg per day of the estrogen lost bone, whereas bone density was maintained in the latter group. Bone loss was proportionately higher in the spine than at the other sites measured. Thus the rate of bone loss from the peripheral cortex did not correlate fully with that from the spine and, hence, was not a reliable indicator of spinal mineral loss. Two of the six women receiving the 0.6 mg dose lost bone. Three women from the placebo group had increased BMD of the spine after taking 0.6 mg per day of the estrogen. This preliminary observation that conjugated estrogens increase bone mineral density in women has been supported by recent data[16] Women 14 days, plus or minus 0.9 years, after menopause, received a daily dose of 0.625 mg of conjugated equine estrogens and cyclic medroxyprogesterone acetate for 12 to 14 days each month and calcium supplements to bring the total calcium intake to approximately 1500 mg per day. Another group of women 13.7 years, plus or minus 1.1 years from menopause received only the calcium supplement. Bone mineral density was measured by dual photon absorptiometry in the lumbar spine and femoral neck. At the end of two years, the bone mineral density of the lumbar spine and femoral neck in the estrogen-treated group increased (5.5% and 1.6% respectively). In the calcium only treated group, bone mineral density decreased at both sites. Although not specifically commented upon, it appears that in six out of 22 patients in the estrogen-treated group, a decrease in bone mineral density occurred, while it increased in some women in the calcium group.

ESTROPIPATE SULFATE

In dose-response studies,[17,18] estropipate (estrone sulfate piperazine) was administered orally in 0.375, 0.75 and 1.5 mg daily, along with 1000 mg of calcium supplement. At the end of two years, subjects receiving either the placebo or the 0.375 mg dose showed a mean decrease (3.6% and 5.1%, respectively) in the bone mineral density of the thoraco-lumbar spine, assessed by quantitative computed tomography. Bone mineral density in those receiving 0.75 mg decreased by 0.8% plus or minuse 1.4%, versus a loss of 3.6% plus or minus 1.5% in the placebo group ($p < 0.1$). Hence some subjects had bone loss on this dose. Subjects taking the 1.5 mg dose increased their bone mineral density by 2%. In the femoral neck, there was a loss in bone density in all groups, except in those receiving 1.5 mg. The minimal dose of estropipate that prevented bone loss from the femoral neck and spine seem to be 1.5 mg and 0.75 mg, respectively, although there were nonresponders to the latter dose.

The greatest difference in bone mineral density between the placebo group and those receiving either 0.75 mg or 1.5 mg of estropipate was at 18 months after beginning the study. Subsequently, the bone mineral density in both estrogen-treated groups declined so that by 24 months, only those on the higher estrogen dose were significantly different from the placebo group. The cause for this decline is unexplained, and it would be pertinent to know what the findings would be in subsequent years. Progestational agents were not given and whether that would have made a difference is speculative. The incidence of endometrial hyperplasia was dose-dependent, being highest in the 1.5 mg group.

During the second phase of this study, women with an intact uterus were also given 10 mg of medoxyprogesterone acetate from days 13 to 25. There seemed to be a dose-response effect on BMD, since women who had previously taken 0.5 mg and were subsequently placed on 1 mg showed further increase in BMD, whereas those previously on the 2 mg dose appeared to lose bone when the dosage was reduced.

MESTRANOL

In a longitudinal study, Lindsay and coworkers[14,16,19–22] examined bone density in a group of women who had undergone bilateral oophorectomy between two months and six years prior to receiving 20 micrograms of mestranol twice daily. However, the amount of mestranol taken by the subjects over the years of study was a rough estimate based on the postcards that patients returned to the pharmacy. Consequently, the findings were based on average dosages for the group (rather than a precise amount taken by each subject), calculated to be between 23 to 25 micrograms per day over the various years of follow-up. Findings from these studies may be summarized as follows: 1) Bone loss in untreated oophorectomized women occurs at a mean rate of 2.7% a year for the first three years, after which it decreases to about 0.7% per year. 2) Mestranol given within two months after bilateral oophorectomy greatly slows bone loss (2.7% versus 0.4% per year). 3) Mestranol begun three or six years after oophorectomy causes an increase in bone mineral density, which is most rapid in the first three years and slows in the ensuing two years. (In those treated six years after the surgical menopause, bone loss continues during the first year.) 4) The level of bone mineral density achieved remains below that present at the time of oophorectomy. 5) The longer the time interval between oophorectomy and beginning estrogen treatment, the slower the rate of increase in bone mineral density. The mean annual change in women treated six years after oophorectomy was 0.3 plus or minus 0.11, compared to 0.57 plus or minus 0.09 in those treated three years after oophorectomy. 6) Discontinuation of estrogen treatment results initially in a rapid rate of bone loss (2.5%) that slows down (0.7% per year), mimicking the course in untreated oophorectomized women. 7) Long-term mestranol therapy (mean of nine years) is accompanied by a slight but significant decrease in bone mineral density. This could represent either a tolerance resistance to estrogen, or an age-related bone loss not influenced by estrogen.

17β ESTRADIOL

Ettinger and coworkers[23] examined BMD of the spine (by dual photon absorptiometry) in postmenopausal women on three dose regimens of micronized 17β estradiol: 0.5 mg, 1 mg and 2 mg per day. All subjects were supplemented with 1500 mg of calcium. Bone mineral density increased by 2% in subjects receiving the 2 mg dose. The minimally effective dose from this study was judged to be 0.5 mg, although it appears that a number of subjects lost bone on this as well as on the 1 mg dose. These findings are somewhat analogous to those reported by Christiansen and colleagues[24] who compared three regimens of estradiol and estriol on the bone mineral density of the distal radius using single-photon absorptiometry. All subjects received cyclic norethisterone (1 mg) and a calcium supplement of 500 mg. The estrogen regimens were: 4 mg estradiol plus 2 mg estriol, or 2 mg estradiol plus 1 mg estriol, or 1 mg estradiol plus 0.5 mg estriol. The results showed a dose-response relationship, with bone density increasing by 1.5% on the highest dose, 0.8% on the medium dose, no change on the lowest dose, and a decrease of 2% in those receiving a placebo. The effects on the spine and femoral neck were not studied.

In their landmark crossover study, Christiansen and coworkers[25] demonstrated that estrogens can prevent and treat osteoporosis associated with menopause. One hundred and fourteen healthy women six months to three years postmenopause were placed on either hormone therapy or a placebo. The former took 4 mg of 17β estradiol and 2 mg of estriol per day from days 1 to 22, and 1 mg of 17β estradiol and 0.5 mg of estriol from days 22 to 28, plus 1 mg of norethisterone on days 13 through 22. All participants were given 500 mg of calcium per day. Two years later, 16 patients in the hormone-treated group were continued on hormone therapy, whereas 19 patients took a placebo. In the placebo group, 19 patients were placed on the hormone regimen, and the remainder continued taking the placebo. Bone mineral density was assessed in the distal part of the forearm. In the hormone-treated group, bone mineral content increased 1.9% after one year, 2.5% after two years, and 3.7% after three years; whereas, when the hormones were withdrawn, bone mineral content fell 2.3% in the ensuing year. In the placebo group, bone mineral content decreased by 1.9% per year and increased by 1.4% in those who were subsequently placed on the hormones.

In contrast to the findings of Lindsay and coworkers,[19,21,22] Christiansen and colleagues[24,25] did not find an accelerated rate of bone loss after estrogen withdrawal. However, the follow-up was for one year, and the findings may have been different in the long term. Other differences between the two studies include: 1) type of menopause (surgical versus 'natural' menopause); 2) type of estrogen (mestranol versus 17β estradiol and estriol); and 3) type of bone studied (third metacarpal bone versus distal forearm).

TRANSDERMAL 17β ESTRADIOL

The effect of three doses of transdermal estrogen on bone markers was evaluated in a double-blind, randomized, placebo-controlled study.[26] Subjects were 40 years or older and had undergone bilateral salpingo-oophorectomy between six weeks and two years before. 17β estradiol was administered transdermally in dosages of 0.025 mg, 0.05 mg, or 0.1 mg per day. Bone mineral content was measured at the mid-radius by single-photon absorptiometry, and in the lumbar spine by dual-photon absorptiometry. At the end of two years, there was a 6.4% decrease in bone mineral density of the spine in the placebo group. In the group on 25 micrograms per day, bone loss in the spine was reduced but not prevented (3.0% loss). The mean bone mineral content in the 50-microgram-per-day group was essentially unchanged (an increase of 0.8% which indicates that a significant number of subjects had lost bone). Subjects receiving the 0.1 mg dose had a significant increase in bone mass. There was bone loss from the radius at all three dosages, but the loss was below that occurring with the placebo.

Lufkin and coworkers[27] looked into the effect of transdermal estradiol on bone density in postmenopausal women with vertebral fractures due to osteoporosis. The women were 47 to 75 years of age and received 0.1 mg of 17β estradiol transdermally daily for 21 days, and 10 mg of medroxyprogesterone acetate (days 11 to 21) for each 28-day cycle. Calcium intake was maintained at about 800 mg per day. Bone densities of the lumbar spine and proximal femur were assessed by dual-photon absorptiometry, and that of the mid-radius by single-photon absorptiometry. At the end of one year, BMD in the placebo group was virtually unchanged; whereas in the estrogen group, the annual rate of change was about 5%. At mid-radius, the mean annual rate was 1% in the estrogen group, compared to −2.6% in the placebo group. The rate of change in the femoral neck (2.6%) was less than that of the femoral trochanter (7.6%). It was not clear why this was so. Eight new vertebral fractures occurred in seven women in the estrogen group, and 20 in 12 women in the placebo group. The mean rate of change in lumbar spine mineral density in the estrogen group was similar in women under or over 65 years of age (5.3% versus 4.4%); that is, the gain in bone mass did not decrease in older women. Increase in bone mass under estrogen treatment seems to continue until a new steady state is reached, at which time the decrease in bone resorption is matched by a decrease in bone formation. Bone mass is maintained, and no further increase occurs. This leveling of the increase in bone density becomes apparent about 18 to 24 months into the treatment, and seems to occur sooner in the lumbar spine than in the femoral neck.[16] This concept is not necessarily contradicted by the findings of the PEPI Trial since, during the latter, BMD was not assessed in the interval between the 12- and 36-month evaluations.

Endometrial hyperplasia occurred in 8% after one year, despite the administration of medroxyprogesterone, and mastodynia in 56% of the women. The reason for this high incidence of endometrial hyperplasia, despite medroxyprogesterone administration, is not forthcoming, but raises important issues regarding the duration and dosage of the progestin treatment in relation to the type and amount of the estrogen.

CONJUGATED EQUINE ESTROGENS

To date, the Postmenopausal Estrogen/Progestin Interventions Trial is the largest placebo-controled, randomized, double-blinded clinical trial that has assessed the effect of estrogen–progestin treatments on spine and hip bone mineral densities. Bone mineral density measurements (BMD) were done by dual-energy X-ray absorptiometry. Postmenopausal women aged 45 to 65 years were assigned to either a placebo or one of four hormone treatment groups, given in 28-day cycles. Conjugated equine estrogens (0.625 mg per day) were given either alone or in conjunction with 2.5 mg per day of medroxyprogesterone acetate. The other two groups received, in addition to the estrogen, either 10 mg per day of medroxyprogesterone acetate or 200 mg per day of micronized progesterone for 12 days each month. At the end of three years, the average loss in bone mineral densities in the spine and hip were 2.8% and 2.2%, respectively, in the placebo group; whereas in the hormone-treated group, bone mineral density increased, on the average by 5.1% and 2.3% at these sites. There was no demonstrable effect attributable to the use of progestins versus the estrogen alone. The preponderance of increase in bone mineral density occurred during the first year, with only 10% to 30% of the increase occurring in the final two years. Bone mineral density loss in both the spine and the hip was greater in women aged 45 to 54 than in those aged 55 to 64 (-4% and -3% versus -2% and -1.6%, respectively). Among those receiving the hormones, the older women gained bone mineral density in their spine (5.9% versus 3.9%) and hip (2.6% versus 2.0%). A high intake of calcium decreased the rate of bone loss in women taking the placebo, but had no apparent effect in those being placed on hormones. Consistent with these findings, bone deposition was slightly greater and bone loss was less in women with no prior history of hormone use, compared to women with a history of hormone use prior to entering the study. The findings from this study showed that 0.625 mg of conjugated equine estrogens taken daily causes an increase in bone mineral density in the spine and hip, and that the addition of a progestational agent had no apparent effect on the amount of bone accrued. Most of the increase in bone mineral density occurred in the first year, and whether the findings at three years represent continued increase (albeit at a slower rate) or a beginning decline from a peak bone mineral density reached sometime during the prior 24 months cannot be ascertained.

Notwithstanding the significance of the Postmenopausal Estrogen/Progestin Interventions Trial, several questions pertaining to hormone replacement therapy remain unanswered. For example; 1) How do the findings from the PEPI Trial apply to other estrogen regimens? 2) Does the (possible) effect of a progestin depend on the type of progestin and/or the type and dose of the estrogen? This is relevant in view of studies showing an added beneficial effect to progestins. 3) How should nonresponders to hormone replacement therapy be managed? Although the PEPI Trial established the progestin regimens to accompany the 0.625 mg of conjugated equine estrogen, the applicability to other estrogens or dosage regimens remains to be seen. We are not aware of studies of comparable magnitude that have addressed this issue with other estrogen formulations.

2. Regimens

Estrogen replacement therapy may be administered in continuous or cyclic regimens. The estrogen preparation most extensively studied in North America, particularly in relation to concomitant progestin administration, is conjugated equine estrogens. In the continuous regimen, 0.625 mg of conjugated equine estrogen and 2.5 mg of MAP p.o. are taken daily. This combination is available commercially as a single tablet. During the first year, 30% to 40% of women can expect various degrees of breakthrough bleeding, the incidence decreasing with the duration of therapy. Nearly 10% of women experience some breakthrough bleeding after the first year.

A second regimen is continuous estrogen/cyclic progestin therapy, where the conjugated equine estrogen is given daily and 5 mg of MPA given on either the first or the last 14 days of every month. The third regimen is cyclic estrogen/progestin, where 0.625 mg of conjugated equine estrogens is given p.o. for 25 days each month, and 5 mg of MPA for the last 14 days of every cycle. Women can expect cyclic, menstrual-like bleeding; with the passage of time, both the amount and frequency of bleeding decreases, some becoming amenorrheic. There is no documented superiority of one regimen over the other, and patient preference is the most material determining factor.

Medroxyprogesterone acetate is the more frequently prescribed progestin in North America. Other progestins (for example, 19-nortestosterone derivatives) have been more popular across the Atlantic. Such progestins are effective in preventing endometrial hyperplasia, but their increased androgenicity make them, in our opinion, not the primary agents of choice.

The progestin with the least androgenic and adverse lipid profile effect is progesterone. Its poor absorbability by the oral route has hindered the use of this compound in hormone replacement regimens. Progesterone is efficiently absorbed from the vagina, and we have liberally used this route in HRT with good results, particularly in women with adverse lipid profiles or intolerable side effects to other progestins. The availability of micronized progesterone has made the oral route an acceptable venue. The precise dosage regimen in relation to the estrogen is still to be determined; however, in the PEPI Trial, an oral dose of 200 mg per day (days 1 through 12) was protective against endometrial hyperplasia. Despite the reliable absorbability of orally administered micronized progesterone, variations among subjects can occur and, until more experience is gained, we recommend that the endometrium be followed closely for possible hyperplasia. In our limited experience, no endometrial hyperplasia has been noted with doses between 200 to 300 mg per day, but a longer follow-up is needed.

Micronized 17β estradiol may be administered in either a continuous or cyclic manner similar to that described for conjugated equine estrogens. The 'standard' dose is 1 mg p.o. per day. Although the accompanying dose of a progestin has not been as extensively studied, we have employed the regimens for conjugated equine estrogens described above and, to date, have found them to be satisfactory.

Estrogens may also be administered by the transdermal route in either a cyclic or continuous manner. Fifty micrograms of 17β estradiol per day is the standard dose. The concomitant dose of progestin has not been as clearly elucidated as that for conjugated equine estrogens; however, the progestin dosage and regimens outlined above appear appropriate and the patient's progress monitored. We do not perform an endometrial biopsy routinely prior to initiating ERT. We do not believe that ERT *per se* represents a valid indication.

The adequacy of estrogen replacement therapy should be monitored both clinically and by laboratory means. As indicated earlier, the absorption of estrogens and progestins can vary in and among individuals. In women who continue to complain of hot flashes, an increase in the estrogen/progestin dosage is recommended. If the complaint continues, other causes should be investigated.

The adequacy of ERT can also be monitored by measuring the plasma level of estradiol. The minimum level should be 50 pg per ml. In addition, bone mineral density of the spine and hip should be assessed at the start of treatment and one or two years later. Subsequent evaluations depend on the direction and adequacy of the change in bone mineral density.

Women on appropriate estrogen replacement therapy may develop symptoms secondary to atrophy in the urogenital system. Such complaints are best handled by local estrogen preparations. Because of their local effect, there is an enhancement of the desired response in comparison to the systemic route. Nonetheless, estrogens are absorbed from the vagina and, in prolonged treatments, endometrial hyperstimulation and other systemic side effects may occur. Patient compliance is also important, particularly in the elderly. Recently, a long-acting vaginal estrogen delivery system containing 2 mg of micronized 17β estradiol, which releases 5 to 10 micrograms per 24 hours of estradiol for a period of three months, has become available. This system appears to be well accepted and effective for the long-term treatment of urogenital disorders in menopaused women.[28,29]

Nonresponders to the 'standard' dosage of ERT

Nonresponders to the standard dose of estrogen therapy have received little attention in the literature, and may be found in either the prevention or the treatment of osteoporosis. The precise magnitude of their number cannot be ascertained from the available data. Confounding factors include: the definition of a nonresponder, the etiology of menopause (surgical versus spontaneous), the reproducibility of the technique for measuring bone loss, the varying techniques and bone sites used in the relevant studies, the often small number and differing ages of women in the various subgroups, and the relatively short duration of follow-up compared to the postmenopausal life expectancy. We have, in our practice, encountered several such situations and are currently assessing the relationship between plasma 17β estradiol levels and the response in bone mineral density, and whether increasing the estrogen dose will correct the problem.

Hassager and coworkers[30] have attempted to address the issue of nonresponders. In their studies carried out over a period of two years, bone mineral content was measured in the distal forearm by single-photon absorptiometry in 171 subjects receiving 17β estradiol and estriol in various doses, estradiol valerate, or percutaneous estrogen cream containing 0.6 mg of 17β estradiol per gram. The authors concluded that the majority of healthy women treated relatively early after their menopause will respond favorably in forearm bone mineral content. However, some will continue to lose bone mineral, but at a slow rate; only 1.2% lost more than 1% a year. Preliminary data on bone mineral density of the spine showed comparable findings. The applicability of these findings to other estrogen regimens and bone sites and the changes beyond two years remains to be determined.

Duration of therapy

Felson and coworkers[31] reviewed records of participants in the Framingham study to assess the effect of prior estrogen treatment on bone density in elderly women. The majority of women had taken a daily dose of 0.625 mg or greater of conjugated estrogen (without a progestin) beginning around the time of their menopause and ending by the age of 65. Bone mineral density was measured by dual-photon absorptiometry in the proximal femur, lumbar spine and femoral neck, and by single-photon absorptiometry in the radius. Women younger than 75 years of age who had taken estrogens for seven or more years had higher bone mineral densities (7.6% to 18.8%) at every site, compared to those who had not taken estrogens. However, in the women 75 years of age or older who had taken estrogen for seven or more years, bone mineral density was higher in the shaft of the radius only. In women younger than 75 years of age, there was a positive correlation between bone mineral density and duration of estrogen therapy, whereas such a correlation was essentially absent in those 75 years of age or older. Thus, although a long-term beneficial effect of estrogen treatment on bone mineral density occurs after discontinuation of the estrogen, bone mineral density will begin to decrease, reaching levels comparable to those in women who had not taken estrogens before. Although there may be age- and estrogen-dependent components of bone loss in women, it appears that estrogen-dependent bone loss lasts well into the postmenopause, and long-term therapy with estrogen could have beneficial values. It is obvious that the longer the duration of estrogen therapy, the longer will be its protective effect. Since most hip fractures occur in women over 75 years of age, it becomes prudent to maintain bone density in this age group, since the risk of hip fracture increases significantly with every decrease of 1 standard deviation in bone mineral density.[32] Prolonged estrogen deficiency may lead to fenestration in the trabecular plates, rendering them thin and friable and, thus, prone to fracture. This change in bone architecture most likely is not responsive to estrogen replacement.

ANDROGEN SUPPLEMENTATION TO HORMONE REPLACEMENT THERAPY

Androgen production declines with menopause. Some consider that the addition of androgens to hormone replacement therapy is beneficial to control recalcitrant vasomotor symptoms (particularly in women on 1.25 mg of conjugated equine estrogens or equivalent), to enhance decreased libido and to ameliorate mood changes. The issue is further complicated by the fact that androgens can have undesirable effects on the lipid profile and androgen-sensitive tissues, such as excessive facial hair growth,[33,34] and adding androgens to ERT appears not to exert a bone-sparing effect.[35] Dow and coworkers[36] studied the effect of estradiol implant versus an estradiol plus testosterone implant in 30 postmenopausal women with decreased libido, and found no significant difference in the outcome. Myers and coworkers found that androgen therapy did not significantly alter mood ratings, sexual behaviors or psychophysiologically measured sexual arousal.[37]

We believe that androgens should not be a routine part of estrogen replacement therapy. Their benefits are debatable and they may cause undesirable side effects. Decreased libido, mood changes, loss of sexual desire and anorgasmia should not automatically be ascribed to the decline of estrogen/androgen production in menopaused women, but should be evaluated in their own right as one would in younger women. Often, such complaints have causes other than the decline in androgen production associated with menopause. Androgen supplements may have a limited role after surgical menopause. We have rarely prescribed androgens, either orally or locally (applied to the genital area). In rare instances where androgens may be considered beneficial, we recommend that the duration of therapy be limited.

HORMONE REPLACEMENT THERAPY AND THE CARDIOVASCULAR SYSTEM

Estrogen replacement therapy lowers the risk for cardiovascular disease in women. Current or prior use of estrogen lowers the risk for the development of coronary disease as well as fatal and nonfatal myocardial infarcts.[38–40] The predominant estrogen was conjugated equine estrogens in doses mostly between 0.625 mg and 1.25 mg per day. There was no increased protection from mortality in acute myocardial infarction with the higher estrogen dose.[39] In a 10-year follow-up study of menopausal women who had received 2.5 mg of conjugated equine estrogens, there was no apparent influence on the risk of heart disease.[41]

In menopausal women, estrogen use, either at the time of angiography or within the preceding three months, is the strongest independent predictor of occlusion scores of the coronaries, and is associated with an 87% reduction in the prevalence of angiographically documented coronary arterial disease.[42,43] Furthermore, estrogens in these women improved survival.

A recent 16-year follow-up from the Nurses Health Study confirms that women who had taken either estrogen alone or with a progestin had a significant decrease in the risk of major coronary heart disease.[44] However, there was no decrease in the risk for stroke among current or past hormone users; there seemed to be an increase in the risk of ischemic stroke among current users. There is no ready explanation of why the findings on stroke from this study differs from that reported in the Leisure World Study[45] or that reported by Finucane and colleagues,[46] which showed a decrease in the mortality from stroke and a decrease in relative risk for stroke among estrogen users. It is anticipated that further observation will clarify this issue.

The cardioprotective effect of estrogens is not negated by the appropriate progestin therapy. Whether estrogens are cardioprotective in women without any evidence of coronary disease is not as firmly established.

The mechanisms by which estrogens beneficially affect the cardiovascular system may be divided into two broad categories: 1) influence on the lipid profile; 2) influence on blood vessels. Briefly summarized, whether given orally, transdermally or vaginally, estrogens increase HDL and lower LDL.[47,48] This occurs sooner with oral versus transdermal estrogens: it may take up to six months for the LDL to reach levels comparable to those achieved after oral estrogens.[49,51] The effect on lipids is blunted by progestins to a degree commensurate with their androgenicity.[52] In the Postmenopausal Estrogen/Progestin Interventions Trial, the average increase in HDL was 5.6 mg/dL with conjugated equine estrogen alone, and between 1.2 and 1.4 mg/dL in combination with a progestin. LDL cholesterol decreased between 14.5 and 17.7 mg/dL.[53]

A possible drawback to estrogen administration is the increase in triglycerides. This effect is initially more pronounced after oral than transdermal administration. The increase in triglycerides can adversely affect the risk of cardiovascular disease.[54] In the PEPI Trial, triblycerides increased between 11 to 13.7 mg/dL.

The beneficial effect of estrogens on the lipid profile explains about 30% to 40% of the protective effects of estrogens on the cardiovascular system. The rest may be mostly accounted for by an effect on blood vessels. In 1969, Abdul-Karim and coworkers demonstrated the vasodilatory effect of 17β estradiol on pulmonary vessels in the rabbit neonate, and ascribed this vasodilatory effect to the increase in acetylcholine.[55–58] Experimentally, 17β estradiol prevents myointimal hyperplasia and collagen biosynthesis by smooth muscle cells, and stimulates prostacycline synthesis as well as exhibiting a calcium channel blocking effect.

HORMONE REPLACEMENT THERAPY AND COGNITIVE FUNCTION IN POSTMENOPAUSAL WOMEN

One of the most exciting developments in recent years is the possible beneficial association between hormone replacement therapy and cognitive function. Although the concept of involutional melancholia as a specific psychiatric disorder associated with menopause has long been rejected, the possible relationship between estrogens and psychological health is still the object of much research.

It is clear that many (not all) women after menopause suffer with varying degrees of severity from problems such as fatigue, nervousness, irritability, headaches and insomnia. Attempts to find a *clear* link between these complaints and estrogen deprivation have failed. The abatement of these symptoms by estrogen replacement has been ascribed to the relief from the hot flush (and its consequences) rather than from a specific effect of the estrogen.[59] More controversial is whether estrogen deficiency induces depression. It is certain that some women do experience mood changes. It is our belief, however, that the major cause of these mood changes is dictated primarily by a woman's own perception of herself, of menopause, or how she is perceived by others and the manner in which she is treated, particularly by those closest to her. Depression is not physiologic but pathologic, and needs to be treated as such, irrespective of age. A recent study did not find a beneficial effect on depression from postmenopausal estrogen use.[60]

The effect of estrogens on cognitive function appears to be highly specific. Estrogens may have beneficial effects on particular aspects of verbal memory, but not on visual memory or attention.[60-63] Emerging also is the tantalizing possibility that estrogen use in postmenopausal women may reduce the incidence and improve the course of dementia. Preliminary findings from the Leisure World cohort study indicate that Alzheimer's disease and related dementia are more common in nonestrogen users than users. The risk of dementia was inversely related to the dose and duration of estrogen.[64,65] Two other studies raise a modicum of hope that estrogen treatment may improve the course of Alzheimer's disease. An open-trial study by Fillit and coworkers[66] showed that 2 mg per day of estradiol for six weeks caused improvement in memory scores in three out of seven women. In the study from Japan, seven women were treated with conjugated equine estrogens (1.25 mg per day) over six weeks, whereas another group of seven women with Alzheimer's disease served as controls. Six of the seven treated women showed appreciable improvement in memory.[67]

Recently, it has been shown that estrogen use in the postmenopausal years is associated with a significant delay in both the onset and frequency of Alzheimer's disease.[68] The authors had a face-to-face interview with each participant. The estrogen they were using was mainly conjugated equine estrogen.

The findings are provocative and should serve as an impetus to randomized, prospective, properly controlled studies to clarify the relationship between postmenopausal estrogen use and dementia.

RISKS OF HORMONE REPLACEMENT THERAPY

Endometrial hyperplasia and endometrial cancer

The prolonged use of estrogens without benefit of progestins increases the risk of both endometrial hyperplasia and endometrial cancer.[69,70] Whitehead and Frazier[71] reported a 30% incidence of endometrial hyperplasia after 18 months of unopposed estrogen use. In the PEPI Trial, the incidence of endometrial hyperplasia in those taking unopposed estrogen was 34% at the end of three years versus 1% in the groups receiving combined estrogen/progestin therapy. Thus, the rate of adenomatous or atypical endometrial hyperplasia in the unopposed estrogen group ran at approximately 10% per year.[72] In the Menopause Study Group report[70] (a one-year, prospective, double-blind study), the incidence of endometrial hyperplasia in women receiving 0.625 mg of conjugated equine estrogens was 20%. Excluding focal cystic hperplasia, the incidence was 8%. Endometrial hyperplasia was absent in those taking the continuous regimen of 0.625 mg of conjugated equine estrogen (CEE) plus 5 mg of medroxyprogesterone acetate (MPA) and in those receiving cyclic 10 mg of MPA for 14 days of each 28-day cycle. In the group on 0.625 CEE plus 2.5 mg of MPA continuous therapy, the incidence of endometrial hyperplasia was less than 1%, whereas in those on 5 mg of MPA for 14 days each 28-day cycle, the incidence was 1%. The incidence of hyperplasia was not statistically different between the groups receiving MPA; nonetheless, it tended to increase with the duration of treatment in both the estrogen-alone and estrogen-progestin groups. Gelfand and Firenze found that the incidence of endometrial hyperplasia is estrogen-dose-related and is reversible under progestin treatment.[73] Conjugated equine estrogens were given in dosages of 0.625 mg or 1.25 mg per day for 25 days each 30-day cycle alone or with 5 mg of MPA on days 15 to 25, inclusive. At the end of six and 12 months, endometrial hyperplasia (persistent proliferative is included in this category) was found in 4% and 0%, respectively, in the group receiving 0.625 mg CEE plus 5 mg MPA, compared to 15% and 30% in the group receiving the conjugated equine estrogen alone. The comparable findings of those receiving 1.25 mg CEE were 17% and 57%, and 0% and 10% in those given additionally the 5 mg MPA. In contrast to the Menopause Group Study, the progestin was used for 11 days in each cycle (versus 14). The minimum dose of MPA received in each cycle in the menopause study group was 70 mg, and the highest was 140 mg; whereas in Gelfand's and Firenze's study, the total dose was 55 mg. Thus, the total dose of MPA seems more important than the type of regimen.[46,70] In another study, both 5 mg and 10 mg of MPA, in conjunction with 1.25 mg of conjugated estrogens, reduced the estrogen receptor concentration of pretreatment levels; whereas 2.5 mg of the MPA did not.[74] However, no significant histologic or biochemical differences in the endometrium were noted after progestin was administered for six days with lower dosage, compared with a higher dosage.[75]

The study by Figueroa-Casas[76] lends further credence to the concept that endometrial hyperplasia may be treatable in combined cyclic hormone replacement therapy regimens. The authors administered 0.625 mg of conjugated equine estrogens for 21 days of each month and MPA (10 mg) from days 12 to 21 to women with a mean postmenopause age of 2.8 years. Six patients had been diagnosed with endometrial hyperplasia prior to treatment, two of whom had the atypical variety. All six reverted to normal endometrium during the course of therapy.

That progestins administered in the appropriate dose reduce the risk for developing endometrial hyperplasia that accompanies the use of estrogens alone is now without question. Since endometrial hyperplasia predisposes to the development of endometrial cancer, one can confidently assume that progestins reduce the risk of endometrial cancer among estrogen users. It is less clear whether the incidence of endometrial cancer among users of combined hormone replacement therapy differs from that of nonusers. Although some studies[77,78] have suggested that the incidence of endometrial cancer is decreased in women on combined therapy, others have either failed to show a difference in the incidence of endometrial cancer or have suggested a slight increase in the relative risk.[79–82] Lack of uniformity in methodology and control for confounding factors may, in part, explain the discrepancy, and the issue merits further controlled studies seeking the answer.

The type of estrogen and progestogen may influence the result as well as does the progestogen/estrogen ratio. The risk of endometrial cancer increases if the dose of estrogen is increased without change in the dose of the progestin. The duration of treatment is also important for endometrial protection. The incidence of endometrial hyperplasia decreased from 4% to 0% when the progestin treatment was extended from 7 to 12 days per month.[71] It appears that the incidence of endometrial pathology is increased if progestins are given for less than 10 days per month.[80]

The risk for endometrial cancer after unopposed estrogen use persists for many years after discontinuation of the estrogen, and the subsequent use of a progestin may not protect fully the endometrium against that risk.[69,83,84] This possibility should be kept in mind, even when such patients are subsequently placed on hormone replacement therapy. This subject has been reviewed recently.[85]

While progestins in women receiving estrogen replacement therapy do protect the endometrium against endometrial hyperplasia and, hence, possibly, cancer, progestins do not eliminate the risk of cancer developing in these women. This finding is consistent with the hypothesis that there could be essentially two types of endometrial cancer – one hormonally related and the other not.[86]

Is the risk of thromboembolic disease increased in women on HRT?

Numerous studies have shown that hormone replacement therapy has little, no, or even a beneficial effect on procoagulant factors. Scarabin and colleagues[87] showed that 17β estradiol (2 mg per day) or conjugated equine estrogens (0.625 mg per day) in conjunction with a progestin caused a significant reduction in plasma fibrinogen and factor VII and a nonsignificant decrease in plasminogen-activating inhibitor; in effect reversing menopause-related changes. In another study, women received either transdermal estradiol (50 micrograms per 24 hours) and 10 mg of MPA daily for 10 days each cycle, or 17β estradiol (2 mg orally for 22 days, 1 mg for six days), and 1 mg of norethindrone acetate for the last 10 days of each cycle. At the end of 12 months there was 56% reduction in tissue factor activity, 30% reduction in tumor necrosis factor, and 35% reduction in thromboxane B2 activity. These beneficial effects took several months to become apparent. No differences were noted between the transdermal or oral routes, and no adverse effect from the progestins was identified.[88] Boschetti and coworkers[89] administered either transdermal estradiol (50 micrograms per day) or 0.625 mg p.o. of conjugated estrogens in a three-week cycle. During the last week, 10 mg of MPA was added. At four months, there was no change in factors VII, VIII, fibrinogen and antithrombin III, compared to pretreatment levels. At 12 months, factor VII, fibrinogen and tissue plasma activating factor did not vary significantly between treatment groups or from baseline, but there was a significant increase in factor VIII in both groups, which the authors contend to be of doubtful clinical relevance. Antithrombin III decreased by 7% to 11%. Since antithrombin III increases in postmenopausal women compared to premenopause, the changes in this factor may be viewed as moving towards premenopausal levels. Similarly, no significant change in fibrinogen was observed in the PEPI Trial.[53] Contrariwise, women receiving a placebo seemed to have more of an increase in fibrinogen than women in any of the active groups.

One may conclude from the above that there should be little concern for an increased risk for thromboembolic disease in women taking hormone replacement therapy. This comforting conclusion has recently been cast in doubt by three clinical studies that have jolted the sanguine view of a lack of increased risk of thromboembolic phenomena with hormone replacement therapy.[90–92] The Nurses Health Study found that current but not past users had a higher risk of pulmonary embolism, but that duration of use had no influence. The Group Health Cooperative Puget Sound Study showed an increase in the relative risk of idiopathic venous thromboembolism, with the possibility that the risk increased with the dose. A higher risk of venous thromboembolism was also shown in the study from Oxford.

Although none of these studies can be considered conclusive, the similarity in findings from diverse institutions certainly gives pause for concern. Admittedly, the studies have their limitations; for example, they were not prospective, randomized or double-blinded. Nonetheless, their findings should be included in the counseling of women about to receive ERT. In the PEPI Trial,[53] no women in the placebo group developed thromboembolic phenomenon, whereas a total of 10 women receiving hormone replacement therapy developed thromboembolic disease (two with pulmonary embolus, two with deep-vein thrombosis and six with superficial phlebitis). Using multiple comparisons, the authors found no statistical differences in the incidence of thromboembolic disease between treatment groups ($p = 0.427$). Examining the data differently, the incidence of thromboembolic events was 1.4% over calculation in the HRT-treated women (10 out of 701). Even if the six cases with superficial phlebitis are excluded, there remain four women with serious thromboembolic disease. The final word has not been written on this subject. At this time, it is our opinion that the benefits of hormone replacement therapy outweigh a possible slight increase in risk for thromboembolic disease. Some women may respond with an exaggerated effect from the estrogen that predisposes them to clot formation. Such women should be investigated for abnormalities in antithrombin III, protein S and protein C. Should such defects be identified, a conscious decision between patient and physician has to be reached on the advisability of hormone replacement therapy. At least in the short run, transdermal estrogen administration may be more appropriate for these patients.[93]

Blood pressure elevation is a theoretical consequence of estrogen replacement therapy. Contrary to the (rare) response in women on oral contraceptives, we have not encountered any elevation of blood pressure in women on hormone replacement therapy. The results from the PEPI Trial showed no change in blood pressure compared to placebos.

BREAST CANCER

One of the most vexing questions of hormone replacement therapy is whether it increases the risk of breast cancer. The true relationship between estrogens (and now progestins) and breast cancer has begged for an answer from the times when women with breast cancer had their pregnancies interrupted and their ovaries removed in an effort to improve prognosis. Regrettably, decades later and numerous studies notwithstanding, the issue is not much clearer. It has gained urgency in view of the increasing number of women eligible for and taking estrogen replacement therapy. The possible link between breast cancer and a woman's age at menarche, first pregnancy or menopause, and the number of ovulatory cycles and pregnancies suggests that endogenous sex hormones may play a role in the etiology of breast cancer. However, the role of endogenous estrogens in the development of breast cancer is still unresolved.[94–96] It has been argued that progestins may reduce the risk of breast cancer. On the other hand, the opposite has also been postulated, based on the fact that mitotic activity in the breast reaches its peak in the luteal phase.

Investigations on possible interaction between hormone replacement therapy and breast cancer are not (with, our knowledge, one possible exception) prospective, double-blinded, randomized studies. In the study by Nachtigall and coworkers[97] women initially received 2.5 mg of conjugated equine estrogens daily and 10 mg of MPA for seven days each month. After 10 years, women who chose to continue hormone replacement therapy took 0.625 mg per day of conjugated estrogen, and 10 days of the progestin each month. These subjects were followed for an additional 12 years. There were six cases of breast cancer in women who had never taken hormones, and none in those who received the hormone treatment.

'Observational' studies have their drawbacks which are often beyond the control of the investigators. For example, the dose and type of estrogen cannot always be precisely determined, rendering comparative analysis between studies difficult. Estradiol valerate has been more commonly used in Europe than in North America, and in dosages that may achieve higher blood levels than those reached with the more commonly used 0.625 mg of conjugated equine estrogens or 1 mg of 17β estradiol. Furthermore, the comparability of the study and control groups can be a factor – for example, the possible influence of prior use of oral contraceptives on the development of breast cancer.[98] In a recent paper, Matthews and coworkers[99] found that postmenopausal women accepting ERT were lighter, better educated, more often White, had lower systolic and diastolic blood pressures, fasting insulin and apoprotein B, a higher level of HDL cholesterol and HDL-2 cholesterol, and engaged in more leisure time and physical activity. While the impact of some of these differences on the incidence of breast cancer may be debatable, their impact on cardiovascular disease is certainly less arguable[100] which illustrates the point as to how much of an observed effect is due to the qualities of the subject and how much can be ascribed to the treatment.

Studies examining a possible link between hormone replacement therapy and breast cancer have been subjected to several meta-analyses. While results from meta-analysis may be helpful, meta-analysis does not correct for any weaknesses or biases in the original studies; further, the studies reviewed reflect the selection criteria of the analyzers.

Recently, it was reported that there was no relationship between breast cancer and postmenopausal hormones in either ever or past users, but that there was a positive correlation between current, long-term users (five years or more) and the frequency of and mortality from breast cancer.[101] Neither the type or dose (0.625 mg versus 1.25 mg CEE) of estrogen or the intake of a progestin affected the risks. Alcohol users on HRT were at higher risk for developing breast cancer than abstainers or alcohol users not on HRT. Other studies have also shown an increase in the risk for breast cancer among estrogen users, with the risk increasing with the duration of use.[102–104] On the other hand, some studies did not evince an increased risk of breast cancer among women taking hormones for five or more years, and suggested that these women tend to have better surveillance and earlier stage disease and a reduced risk in mortality from breast cancers.[45,105–108] Furthermore, women beginning estrogen replacement at a young age (under 40) seem to have a decreased risk for breast cancer.[109] There is no ready explanation for this rather unique finding but, for an argument's sake, one may hypothesize that the earlier menopause shortened the time the breast was exposed to the endogenous hormones and that the amount of estrogens taken (per month) during hormone replacement therapy is significantly below that produced in a normal menstrual cycle. Another study failed to show a clear increase in risk in breast cancer among either estrogen-alone or estrogen-plus-progestin users, even when taken for longer than five years.[110] Any increased risk for breast cancer in hormone users seemed to be exclusively in lean women. Dupont and Page[111] concluded that doses of 0.625 mg per day or less of conjugated estrogens are not associated with an incrased risk for breast cancer.

In examining the possible relationship between hormone replacement therapy and breast cancer, it is important to factor in the time interval between beginning treatment and the diagnosis of breast cancer. Women on hormone replacement therapy tend to have denser breasts on mammography, which reduces both the specificity and sensitivity of the mammogram and may lead to a proportionately higher diagnosis of breast cancer after apparently normal mammograms.[112]

Does hormone replacement therapy adversely affect the prognosis of women with breast cancer?

We are unaware of any randomized, prospective studies that have focused on this issue. It is our current opinion that the available evidence does not indicate that exogenous estrogens in the dosages used for hormone replacement therapy influence the outcome of at least most of the patients with breast cancer. As in all aspects of medicine, full disclosure and patient cooperation and unequivocal understanding of the issues is necessary. However, the potential medicolegal implications of administering estrogens to women with a history of breast cancer often serves as a deterrent. This subject has recently been reviewed.[113–115] With discovery of BRCA1 and BRCA2 genes, new questions could arise regarding the use of HRT for women carrying those genes.

Clinicians concerned about the possible relationship of ERT and breast cancer may consider administering estrogens vaginally for those patients with intolerable symptoms of vaginal atrophy. Estrogens are absorbed quite efficiently from the vagina, particularly from an atrophic mucosa. With vaginal cornification, the amount absorbed decreases.

Small amounts of estrogen administered intravaginally twice a week may be sufficient for the vaginal mucosa to be maintained with little systemic absorption. The amount absorbed can be monitored by measuring the estrogen blood levels.[116,117]

In conclusion, a definitive answer cannot be given to the question; 'Does hormone replacement therapy affect the risk for breast cancer?' We believe that if there is an increase in risk, its magnitude is small and must be factored into the equation of the risk/benefit ratio of hormone replacement therapy. This subject has been reviewed recently.[118] There are now good alternate medications to treat osteoporosis associated with the menopause. However, the advantages of hormone replacement therapy extend beyond their beneficial effect on osteoporosis, and the range of potential benefits keeps expanding, such as dental health,[119] and colon cancer,[120] among others.

REFERENCES

1 Kuiper GG, Enmark E, Pelto-Huikko M, Nilsson S, Gustafsson JA: Cloning of a hoval receptor expressed in rat prostate and ovary. *Proc Natl Acad Sci USA* 93: 5925–5930, 1996.

2 Yang NN, Venugopalan M, Hardikar S, Glasebrook A: Identification of an estrogen response element activated by metabolites of 17β-estradiol and raloxifene. *Science* 273: 1222–1225, 1996.

3 Szego C, Pietras RJ: Lysosomal functions in cellular activation, propogation of the actions of hormones and other effectors. In Bourne GH, Danielli JF, Jean JW eds, *International Review of Cytology*, 88. New York: Academic Press, 1984.

4 Aronica SM, Craus WL, Katzenellenbogen BS: Estrogen action via the cAMP signalling pathway: Stimulation of adenylate cyclase and cAMP regulated gene transcription. *Proc Natl Acad Sci* 91: 8517, 1994.

5 Hammond CB, Maxon WS: Current status of estrogen therapy for the menopause. *Fert Steril* 37: 5–25, 1982.

6 Maschak CA, Rogeno L, Dozono-Takano R, Eggena P, Nakamura RM, Brenner PF, Mishell DR: Comparison of pharmacodynamic properties of various estrogen formulations. *Am J Obstet Gynecol* 144: 511–918, 1982.

7 Brinton RD: Equilin, a major component of premarin, increases the growth of neurons from the cerebral cortex. *J Soc Gynecol Inv* 13 (Suppl): 70A, 1996.

8 Subiah MTR, Kessel B, Agrawal M, Rajan R, Abplanalp W, Rymaszewski Z: Antioxidant potential of specific estrogens on lipid peroxidation. *J Clin Endocrinol Metab* 77: 1095–1097, 1993.

9 Albright F, Bloomberg E, Smith PH: Postmenopausal osteoporosis. *Transaction of the Association of American Physicians* 55: 298–305, 1940.

10 Albright F, Smith PH, Richardson AM: Postmenopausal osteoporosis. *JAMA* 116: 246–274, 1941.

11 Abdul-Karim RW, Prior JT, Nesbitt REL: The influence of maternal estrogens on fetal bone development in the rabbit. *Obstet Gynecol* 31: 346, 1968.

12 Abdul-Karim RW, Prior JT, Marshall LD: Spontaneous reversibility of fetal pathologic bone development under the influence of an antiestrogenic compound. *Reprod Med* 1: 397, 1968.

13 Abdul-Karim RW, Marshall LD: The influence of ethamoxytriphetol on the collagen and calcium contents of the femurs of rabbit fetuses. *Toxicol Appl Pharmacol* 15: 185, 1969.

14 Lindsay R, Hart DM, Clark DM: The minimum effective dose for the prevention of postmenopausal bone loss. *Am J Obstet Gynecol* 63: 759–763, 1984.

15 Genant HK, Cann CE, Ettinger B, Gordon GS: Quantitative computed tomography of vertebral spongiosa: a sensitive method for detecting early bone loss after oophorectomy. *Ann Inter Med* 97: 699–705. 1982.

16 Lindsay R, Tohme JF: Estrogen treatment of patients with established postmenopausal osteoporosis. *Obstet Gynecol* 76: 290–295, 1990.

17 Harris ST, Genant HK, Baylink DJ, Gallagher JC, Karp SK, McConnell MA, Green EM, Stoll RW: The effects of estrone (Ogen) on spinal bone density of postmenopausal women. *Arch Int Med* 151: 1980–1984, 1991.

18 Gallagher JC, Baylink D: Effect of estrone sulfate on bone mineral density of the femoral neck and spine. *J Bone Mineral Res* 5: (Suppl)S275, 1990.

19 Lindsay R, Hart DM, Aitken JM, MacDonald EB, Clarke AC: Long-term prevention of postmenopausal osteoporosis by estrogen. Evidence for an increased bone mass after delayed onset of estrogen treatment. *Lancet* 1038–1041, 1976.

20 Aitken JM, Hart DM, Lindsay R: Estrogen replacement therapy for the prevention of osteoporosis after oophorectomy. *Br Med J* 8: 515–518, 1973.

21 Lindsay R, Hart DM, MacLean A, Clark AC, Kraszewski A, Garwood J: Bone response to termination of estrogen treatment. *Lancet* 1325–1327, 1978.

22 Lindsay R, Hart DM, Forrest C, Baird C: Prevention of spinal osteoporosis in oophorectomized women. *Lancet* 29: 1151–1153, 1980.

23 Ettinger B, Genant HK, Stiger P, Madvig P: Low-dose micronized 17–Beta estradiol prevents bone loss in postmenopausal women. *Am J Obstet Gynecol* 166: 479–488, 1992.

24 Christiansen C, Christiansen MS, Larsen NE, Transbol I: Pathophysiological mechanisms of estrogen effect on bone metabolism. Dose-response relationships in early postmenopausal women. *J Clin Endocrinol Metab* 55: 1124–1130, 1982.

25 Christiansen V, Christiansen MS, Transbol IB: Bone mass in postmenopausal women after withdrawal of estrogen/progestagen replacement therapy. *Lancet* 28: 459–461, 1981.

26 Field CS, Ory SJ, Herrmann RR, Howard L, Judd HL, Riggs BL: Preventive effects of transdermal beta estradiol on osteoporotic changes after surgical menopause: a two-year placebo-controlled trial. *Am J Obstet Gynecol* 168: 114–121, 1993.

27 Lufkin EG, Eahner H, O'Fallon WM, *et al.*: Treatment of postmenopausal osteoporosis with transdermal estrogen. *Ann Intern Med* 117: 1–9, 1992.

28 Ayton RA, Darling GM, Murkies AL, *et al.*: A comparative study of safety and efficacy of continuous low-dose estradiol released from a vaginal ring compared with conjugated equine estrogen vaginal cream in the treatment of postmenopausal urogenital atrophy. *Br J Obstet Gynecol* 103: 351–358, 1996.

29 Henriksson L, Stjernquist M, Boquist L, *et al.*: A one-year multicenter study of efficacy and safety of a continuous, low-dose, estradiol-releasing vaginal ring (Estring) in postmenopausal women with symptoms and signs of urogenital aging. *Am J Obstet Gynecol* 174: 85–92, 1996.

30 Hassager C, Jenson SB, Christiansen C: Non-responders to hormone replacement therapy for the prevention of postmenopausal bone loss: Do they exist? *Osteoporosis International* 4: 36–41, 1994.

31 Felson DT, Zhang Y, Anderson JJ, *et al.*: The effect of postmenopausal estrogen therapy on bone density in elderly women. *N Eng J Med* 329: 1141–1146, 1993.

32 Cummings SR, Black DM, Nevitt MC, *et al.*: Bone density at various sites for prediction of hip fractures. *Lancet* 341: 72–75, 1993.

33 Urman B, Pride SM, Ho Yeun BH: Elevated serum testosterone, hirsutism and virilism associated with combined androgen-estrogen hormone replacement therapy. *Obstet Gynecol* 77: 595–598, 1991.

34 Hickok LR, Toomey C, Speroff L: A comparison of esterified estrogens with and without methyltestosterone: Effects on endometrial histology and serum lipoproteins in postmenopausal women. *Obstet Gynecol* 82: 919–924, 1993.

35 Garnet T, Studd J, Wastson N, Savvas M: The effects of plasma estradiol levels on increases in

vertebral and femoral bone density following therapy with estradiol and estradiol with testosterone implants. *Obstet Gynecol* 79: 968–972, 1992.

36 Dow MTG, Hart DM: Hormonal treatments of sexual unresponsiveness in postmenopausal women. *Br J Obstet Gynecol* 90: 361–366, 1983.

37 Myers LS, Dixon J, Morrissette M, *et al.*: Effects of estrogen, androgen and progestin on sexual psychophysiology and behavior in postmenopausal women. *J Clin Endo Metab* 70: 1124–1131, 1990.

38 Stampfer M, Willette WC, Colditz GA, Rosner B, Speizer FE, Hennekens CH: A prospective study of postmenopausal estrogen therapy and coronary heart disease *N Eng J Med* 313: 1044–1049, 1985.

39 Henderson BE, Paganini-Hill A, Ross RK: Estrogen replacement therapy and protection from acute myocardial infarction. *Am J Obstet Gynecol* 159: 312–317, 1988.

40 Sullivan JM, Vander Zwag R, Lemp GF, *et al.*: Postmenopausal estrogen use and coronary atherosclerosis. *Ann Intern Med* 108: 358–363, 1988.

41 Nachtigall LE, Nachtigall RH, Nachtigall R, Beckman M: Estrogen replacement therapy II: A prospective study in relation to carcinoma and cardiovascular and metabolic problems. *Obstet Gynecol* 54: 74–79, 1979.

42 Gruchow HW, Anderson AJ, Barboriak JJ, *et al.*: Postmenopausal use of estrogen and occlusion of coronary arteries. *Am Heart J* 115: 954–963, 1988.

43 Hong MK, Romm PA, Reagan K, *et al.*: Effects of estrogen replacement therapy on serum lipid values and angiographically defined coronary disease in postmenopausal women. *Am J Cardiol* 69: 176–178, 1992.

44 Grodstein F, Stampfer MJ, Manson JE, Colditz GA, Willett WC, Rosner B, Speizer FE, Hennekens CH: Postmenopausal estrogen and progestin use and the risk of cardiovascular disease. *N Engl J Med* 335: 453–461, 1996.

45 Henderson BE, Paganini-Hill A, Ross RK: Decreased mortality in users of estrogen replacement therapy. *Arch Int Med* 151: 75–78, 1991.

46 Finucane FF, Madans JH, Bush TL, Wolf PH, Kleinman JC: Decreased risk of stroke among postmenopausal hormone users. *Arch Intern Med* 153: 73–79, 1993.

47 Bush TL, Miller VT: Effect of pharmacologic agents used during menopause: Impact on lipids and lipoproteins. In Mishell DR, ed. *Menopause Physiology and Pharmacology*. Chicago: Mosby Yearbook Medical Publishers, Inc. 1987, pp. 187–208.

48 Gobelsmann V, Maschak A, Mishell DR: Comparison of hepatic oral and vaginal administration to ethinyl estradiol. *Am J Obstet Gynecol* 151: 868–877, 1985.

49 Tikkanen MJ, Nikkila EA, Kussi T, Sipinen S: High density lipoprotein-2 and hepatic lipase: Reciprocal changes produced by estrogen and norgestrel. *J Clin Endocrinol Metabol* 54: 1113–1117, 1982.

50 Tikkanen JM, Nikkila EA, Kussi T, Sipinen S: Different effects of two progestins on plasma HDL and post-heparin hepatic lipase activity. *Atherosclerosis* 40: 365–369, 1981.

51 Walsh BW, Schiff I, Rosner B, Greenberg L, Ravnikar V, Sacks FM: Effect of postmenopausal estrogen replacement on the concentration and metabolism of plasma lipoproteins. *N Eng J Med* 325: 1196–1204, 1991.

52 Samaan SA, Crawford MH: Estrogen and cardiovascular function after menopause. *J Am Coll Cardiol* 26(6): 1403–1410, 1995.

53 The Writing Group: Postmenopausal estrogen/progestin intervention trial. Effect of estrogen/progestin regimen on heart disease risk factors in postmenopausal women. *JAMA* 273: 199–208, 1995.

54 Bass KM, Newschafer CJ, Klag MJ, Bush TL: Plasma lipoprotein level as predictor of death in women. *Arch Intern Med* 153: 2209–2216, 1993.

55 Abdul-Karim RW, Prior JT: The influence of estrogens on the lung vasculature of the premature rabbit neonate. *Reprod Med* 11: 140, 1969.

56 Abdul-Karim RW, Marshall LD, Nesbitt REL; The influence of 17β estradiol on the acetylcholine content of the lung in the rabbit neonate. *Am J Obstet Gynecol* 107: 641, 1970.

57 Abdul-Karim RW, Drucker M, Jacobs RD: The influence of estradiol-17β on cholinesterase activity in the lung. *Am J Obstet Gynecol* 108: 1098–1101, 1970.

58 Abdul-Karin RW, Erhar K, Drucker M: The dose-time relationship of estradiol-17β and lung cholinesterase. *Am J Obstet Gynecol* 110: 424–426. 1971.

59 Campbell S, Whitehead M: Estrogen therapy and premenopausal syndrome. *Clin Obstet Gynecol* 4: 31–47, 1977.

60 Palinkas LA, Barrett-Connor E: Estrogen use and depressive symptoms in postmenopausal women. *Obstet Gynecol* 80: 30–36, 1992.

61 Barret-Connor E, Kritz-Silverstein D: Estrogen replacement therapy and cognitive function in older women. *JAMA* 260: 2637–2641, 1993.

62 Kampen DL, Sherwin BB: Estrogen use and verbal memory in healthy postmenopausal women. *Obstet Gynecol* 83: 979–983, 1994.

63 Sherwin BB, Phillips S: Estrogen and cognitive functioning in surgically menopausal women. *Ann NY Acad Sci* 592: 475–492, 1990.

64 Paganini-Hill A, Henderson VW: Estrogen deficiency and risk of Alzheimer's disease in women. *Am J Epidemiol* 140: 256–261, 1994.

65 Henderson VW, Paganini-Hill A, Emanuel CK, Dunn ME: Estrogen replacement therapy in older women. *Arch Neurol* 896–900, 1994.

66 Filit H, Weinreb H, Cholse I, *et al.*: Observations in a preliminary open trial of estradiol therapy for senile dementia – Alzheimer's type. *Psychoneuroendocrinology* 11: 337–345, 1986.

67 Recker RR, Savill PD, Heaney RP: Effect of estrogen and calcium carbonate on bone loss in postmenopausal women. *Ann Intern Med* 87: 649–655, 1977.

67 Honjo H, Ogino Y, Naithoh K, *et al.*: In vivo effects by estrone sulphate on central nervous system – senile dementia (Alzheimer's type). *J Steroid Biochem* 34: 521–525, 1989.

68 Tang MX, Jacobs D, Stern Y, Marder K, Schofield P, Gurland B, Andrews H, Mayeux R: Effects of estrogen during menopause on risk and age of onset of Alzheimer's. *Lancet* 348: 429–432, 1996.

69 Shapiro S, Kelly JP, Rosenberg L, Kaufman DW, *et al.*: Risk of localized and widespread endometrial cancer in relation to recent and discontinued use of conjugated estrogens. *N Eng J Med* 313: 969–972, 1985.

70 Woodruff JD, Pickar JH: For the menopause study group. Incidence of endometrial hyperplasia in postmenopausal women taking conjugated estrogen (Premarin) with medroxyprogesterone acetate or conjugated estrogens alone. *Am J Obstet Gynecol* 170: 1213–1223, 1994.

71 Whitehead MI, Fraser D: Controversies concerning the safety of estrogen replacement therapy. *Am J Obstet Gynecol* 156: 1313–1322, 1987.

72 Effects of hormone therapy on bone mineral density. Results from the Postmenopausal/Progestin Interventions (PEPI) trial. *JAMA* 276: 1389–1396, 1996.

73 Gelfand MM, Ferenczy A: A prospective one-year study of estrogen and progestin in postmenopausal women: Effects on the endometrium. *Obstet Gynecol* 74: 398–402, 1989.

74 Gibbons WE, Moyer LD, Lobo RA, Roy S, Michel DR: Biochemical and histologic effects of sequential estrogen/progestogen therapy on the endometrium of postmenopausal women. *Am J Obstet Gynecol* 154: 456–461, 1986.

75 Whitehead MI, Townsend PT, Tryse-Davies J, Ryder TA, King RJ: Effect of estrogen and progestogen on the biochemistry and morphology of the postmenopausal endometrium. *N Eng J Med* 305: 1599–1605, 1981.

76 Figueroa-Casas PR, Schlaen I: Sequential use of conjugated estrogen and medroxyprogesterone in the climacteric syndrome: clinical and histological findings. *Maturitas* 9: 309–313, 1988.

77 Gambrell RD Jr: The menopause: Benefits and risks of estrogen/progestogen replacement therapy. *Fertil Steril* 37: 457–474, 1982.

78 Nachtigall LE, Nachtigall RH, Nachtigall RD, Beckmann EM: Estrogen replacement therapy – I. A 10-year prospective study in relationship to osteoporosis. *Obstet Gynecol* 53: 277–281, 1979.

79 Person J, Adami HO, Bergkvist L, *et al.*: Risk of endometrial cancer after treatment with estrogens alone or in conjunction with progestogens. *Br Med J* 298: 147–151, 1989.

80 Voigt LF, Weiss NS, Chu J, Daling JR, McKnight B, Van Belle G: Progestogen supplementation of exogenous estrogens and risk of endometrial cancer. *Lancet* 338: 274–277, 1991.

81 Jick SS, Walker AM, Jick H: Estrogens, progesterone and endometrial cancer. *Epidemiol* 4: 20–24, 1993.

82 Brinton LA, Hoover RN: The endometrial cancer collaboration group. Estrogen replacement therapy and endometrial cancer risk. Unresolved issues. *Obstet Gynecol* 81: 265–271, 1993.

83 Kennedy DL, Baum C, Forbes MB: Non-contraceptive estrogens and progestins. Use patterns over time. *Obstet Gynecol* 65: 441–446, 1985.

84 McGonigle KF, Karlan BY, Barbuto DA, *et al.*: Development of endometrial cancer in women on estrogen and progestin HRT. *Gynecol Oncol* 55: 126–132, 1994.

85 Grady D, Gebretsadik T, Kerlikowske K, Ernster V, Petitti D: Hormone replacement therapy and endometrial cancer risk: A meta-analysis. *Obstet Gynecol* 85: 304–313, 1995.

86 Bokhman JV: Two pathogenic types of endometrial carcinoma. *Gynecol Oncol* 15: 10–17, 1983.

87 Scarabin PY, Plu-Burrau G, Bana L, *et al.*: Haemostatic variables and menopausal status: Influence of hormone replacement therapy. *Thromb Haemost* 70: 584–587, 1993.

88 Aune B, Oian P, Omsjo I, Osterud Bjarne: Hormone replacement therapy reduces the reactivity of monocytes and platelets in whole blood – A beneficial effect on atherogenesis and thrombus formation? *Am J Obstet Gynecol* 173(6): 1816–1820, 1995.

89 Boschetti C, Cortellaro M, Nencioni T, Bertolli V, Della Volpe A, Zanussi G: Short- and long-term effects of hormone replacement therapy (transdermal estradiol vs. oral conjugated equine estrogens, combined with medroxyprogesterone acetate) on blood coagulation factors in post-menopausal women. *Thromb Res* 62: 1–8, 1991.

90 Daly E, Vessey MP, Hawkins MM, Carson JL, Gough P, Marsh S: Risk of venous thromboembolism in users of hormone replacement therapy. *Lancet* 348: 977–980, 1996.

91 Jick H, Derby LE, Myers MW, Vasilakis C, Newton KM: Risk of hospital admission for idiopathic venous thromboembolism among users of postmenopausal oestrogens. *Lancet* 348: 981–983, 1996.

92 Grodstein F, Stampfer MJ, Goldhaber SZ, Manson JE, Colditz GA, Speizer FE, Willett WC, Hennekens CH: Prospective study of exogenous hormones and risk of pulmonary embolism in women. *Lancet* 348: 983–987, 1996.

93 Badaway SZA, Abdul-Karim RW: Does protein C deficiency contraindicate the use of estrogen? *Collected Letters: Int Corresp Soc Obstet Gynecol* 35(8): 5–6, 1994.

94 Abdul-Karim RW, Badaway SZA, Maini S: Natural hormone replacement therapy: Does use of estriol prevent breast cancer? *Collected Letters: Int Corresp Soc Obstet Gynecol* 38(1): 3–4, 1997.

95 Toniolo PG, Levitz M, Jacquotte AZ, Banerjee S, Koenig KL: A prospective study of endogenous estrogens and breast cancer in postmenopausal women. *J Natl Can Inst* 87: 190–197, 1995.

96 Helzlsouer KY, Alberg AJ, Bush TL, *et al.*: A prospective study of endogenous hormones and breast cancer. *Can Det Prev* 18: 79, 1994.

97 Nachtigall MJ, Smilen SW, Nachtigall RAD, Nachtigall RH, Nachtigall LI: Incidence of breast cancer in a 22-year study of women receiving estrogen–progestogen replacement therapy. *Obstet Gynecol* 80: 827–830, 1992.

98 Collaborative group on hormonal factors in breast cancer: Breast cancer and hormonal contraceptives: Collaborative reanalysis of individual data on 53,297 women with breast cancer and 100,239 women without breast cancer from 54 epidemiological studies. *Lancet* 347: 1713–1727, 1996.

99 Matthews KA, Kuller HK, Wing RR, Meilahn EN, Plantinga P: Prior to use of estrogen replacement therapy, are users healthier than non-users? *Am J Epidemiol* 143: 971–978, 1996.

100 Grodstein F: Invited commentary: Can selection bias explain the cardiovascular benefits of estrogen replacement therapy? *Am J Epidemiol* 143: 979–982, 1996.

101 Colditz GA, Hackenson SE, Hunter DJ: Use of estrogens and progestogens and the risk of breast cancer in postmenopausal women. *N Eng J Med* 332: 1589–1593, 1995.

102 Risch HA, Howe GR: Menopausal hormone usage and breast cancer in Saskatchewan: A record linkage cohort study. *Am J Epidemiol* 139: 670–683, 1994.

103 Schairer C, Byrne C, Keyl PM, *et al.*: Menopausal estrogen and estrogen progestin replacement therapy and risk of breast cancer. *Cancer Causes Control* 5: 491–500, 1994.

104 La Vecchia C, Negri E, Franceschi S, *et al.*: Hormone replacement treatment and breast cancer risk: A cooperative Italian study. *Br J Cancer* 72: 244–248, 1995.

105 Strickland DM, Gambrell RD Jr, Butzin CA, Strickland K: The relationship between breast cancer survival and prior menopausal estrogen use. *Obstet Gynecol* 80: 400–404, 1992.

106 Bergkvist L, Adami HO, Persson I, Bergstrom R, Krusemo UB: Prognosis after breast cancer diagnosis in women exposed to estrogen and estrogen and progestogen replacement therapy. *Am J Epidemiol* 130: 221–227, 1989.

107 Stanford JL, Weiss MD, Voight LF, Daling JR, Habel LA, Rossing MA: Combined estrogen and progestin hormone replacement therapy in relation to risk of breast cancer in middle aged women. *JAMA* 247: 137–142, 1995.

108 Shuurman AG, Van Den Brandt PA, Goldbohm RA: Exogenous hormone use and the risk of postmenopausal breast cancer. Results from the Netherlands cohort study. *Cancer Causes Control* 6: 416, 1996.

109 Willis DB, Calle EE, Miracle-McHill HL, *et al.*: Estrogen replacement therapy and risk of fatal breast cancer in a prospective cohort of postmenopausal women in the United States. *Cancer Causes Control* 7: 449, 1996.

110 Newcomb PA, Longnecker MP, Storer BE, *et al.*: Long-term hormone replacement therapy and risk of breast cancer in postmenopausal women. *Am J Epidemiol* 142: 788–795, 1995.

111 Dupont WD, Page DL: Menopausal estrogen replacement therapy and breast cancer. *Arch Int Med* 151: 67–72, 1991.

112 Laya MB, Larson EB, Tapilin SH, White E: Effect of estrogen replacement therapy on the specificity and sensitivity of screening mammography. *J Natl Can Inst* 88: 643–649, 1996.

113 Di Sïa PJ: Estrogen replacement therapy for the breast cancer survivor. *J Soc Gynecol Invest* 3: 57–59, 1995.

114 Creasman WT: Estrogen replacement therapy: Is previously treated cancer a contraindication? *Obstet Gynecol* 77: 308–312, 1991.

115 Vassilopoulou-Sellin R, Klein MJ: Estrogen replacement therapy after treatment for localized breast carcinoma: Patient responses and options. *Cancer* 78: 1043–1048, 1996.

116 Nillson K, Heimer G: Low-dose estradiol in the treatment of urogenital estrogen deficiency. A pharmacokinetic and pharmacodynamic study. *Maturitas* 15: 121–127, 1992.

117 Rigg LA, Hermann H, Yen SSC: Absorption of estrogens from vaginal cream. *N Eng J Med* 298: 195–198, 1978.

118 Speroff L: Postmenopausal hormone therapy and breast cancer. *Obstet Gynecol* 87: 44s–54s, 1996.

119 Paganini-Hill A: The benefits of estrogen replacement therapy on oral health: The Leisure World cohort. *Arch Intern Med* 155: 2325–2329, 1995.

120 Newbomb PA, Storer BE: Postmenopausal hormone use and risk of large-bowel cancer. *J Natl Cancer Inst* 87: 1067–1071, 1995.

13

Estrogen therapy in breast and endometrial cancer survivors

MARY J CUNNINGHAM AND GREGORY R HARPER

INTRODUCTION

As the benefits of hormone replacement therapy (HRT) have become more clearly defined, the treatment with HRT of the large group of women who are survivors of hormone-dependent cancers becomes a more pressing issue. Each year over 200,000 women are diagnosed with hormonally dependent cancers, primarily carcinomas of the breast and endometrium. More than 80% of these patients can expect long-term survival.[1] While these carcinomas have been classified as 'hormonally dependent', the true effect of HRT on recurrence rates and overall survival remains unclear. It is clear that cancer survivors are likely to experience the same benefits with HRT as women who have not had cancer with regard to decrease in ischemic heart disease, osteoporosis, Alzheimer's disease, colon carcinoma, relief of vasomotor symptoms and improvement in overall quality of life. It is against this background of clearly defined benefits and uncertain risks that women and their physicians are forced to make decisions regarding therapy.

ENDOMETRIAL CANCER SURVIVORS AND MENOPAUSE

Endometrial carcinoma is the fourth most common cancer in women in the U.S., and is the most common cause of female genital tract malignancy. Most women are menopausal at the time of diagnosis. Since the optimal therapy for endometrial carcinoma begins with total abdominal hysterectomy and bilateral salpingoophorectomy, all women are menopausal following initial therapy. Up to 25% of patients with endometrial carcinoma are pre-menopausal and develop acute onset of menopause postoperatively. Those with disease confined to the uterine corpus enjoy long-term survival, with recurrence rates of less than 10%.[2] These women remain subject to the same risks of estrogen deprivation as those without malignancies, leading to the consideration of estrogen replacement therapy (ERT) in this population.

HORMONE REPLACEMENT THERAPY AND ENDOMETRIAL CANCER RISK

The relationship of estrogen to the development of endometrial carcinoma has been clearly defined. The association between unopposed exogenous estrogen therapy and an increased risk of endometrial carcinoma was first described in the mid 1970s. Unopposed estrogen use is associated with a relative risk of endometrial carcinoma of 2.3 (confidence interval 2.1–2.5).[3] This increased risk rises with increasing duration of use and persists for at least five years after discontinuation of therapy. More than 10 years of unopposed estrogen use has been associated with an almost ten-fold increase in the risk of developing endometrial carcinoma. Endometrial cancers that develop in women who are taking estrogens have been found to be lower grade, earlier stage, and have less risk of myometrial invasion when compared with cancers in women who are not taking hormones.[4] Despite this relatively favorable pattern of disease, the risk of death from endometrial cancer is two to four times higher in users of unopposed estrogens.[5–8]

Endogenous states which lead to high levels of unopposed estrogen such as chronic anovulation have also been associated with an increased risk of endometrial carcinoma. A common cause of increased endogenous estrogen is obesity, which results in increased peripheral conversion of androstenedione to estrone. Indeed, women who are 30 pounds over ideal body weight have a threefold increase in risk of endometrial cancer, while those who are 50 pounds over ideal body weight have been described to have a tenfold increase in risk.[2] Estrogen-producing ovarian tumors such as granulosa cell tumors have also been associated with a high risk of endometrial cancer. Thus, the relationship of increased unopposed estrogen levels to the development of endometrial carcinoma is well documented.

The protective effect of progestins in patients who are taking ERT has also been investigated. The dose and duration of progestin use appear to be important in decreasing the risk of ERT. Both cyclic therapy using 10 or more days of progestin per month and combined continuous therapy using both estrogen and progestins daily have odds ratios close to 1.[9] Studies have differed in their findings, however, with cohort studies favoring a protective effect while case-control studies show a slight increase in risk.[3]

ESTROGEN THERAPY AND ENDOMETRIAL CANCER SURVIVORS

Because of the clearly defined relationship of exogenous ERT with the development of endometrial carcinoma, physicians and patients alike have been reluctant to consider ERT following treatment for endometrial carcinoma. Indeed, even the package insert for Premarin states that 'you should not take estrogens if you have ever had cancer of the breast or uterus.'[10] Should this be the case? Of concern is the possibility of an increase in recurrence rate or a decrease in survival among patients who are treated with estrogens.

Though prospective data are lacking, there are retrospective studies examining the effect of HRT on patients who have been previously treated for early-stage endometrial carcinoma. The three series published to date encompass a total of 153 treated patients and 297 controls.[11–13] Though most patients were clinical or surgical Stage 1 and thus at low risk of recurrence, some patients with positive cytology and positive pelvic lymph nodes were included. Most patients were treated with estrogen alone without progesterone. The time from treatment for endometrial carcinoma to initiation of ERT was less than two years. This is an important factor since 80% of recurrences of endometrial carcinoma will occur in the first two years following therapy.[2] Beginning therapy early not only avoids selection bias such as selecting out patients less likely to recur, but also avoids the bone loss and other sequellae of prolonged estrogen deprivation.

Two series examined the effects of HRT on patients with clinical Stage 1 endometrial carcinoma. Creasman and colleagues demonstrated a recurrence rate of 2.1% in patients treated with ERT versus 14.9% in those not treated with estrogen.[11] The treatment groups were somewhat biased, however, with patients receiving estrogen having fewer poor prognostic indicators. It is notable that HRT was not associated with a marked increase in recurrence rate. In addition, deaths due to intercurrent disease occurred in 5.7% of patients who were not treated with estrogen while no patients treated with estrogen therapy died of intercurrent disease. Lee and coworkers likewise demonstrated no significant difference in recurrence risks between patients treated with estrogen versus no estrogen.[12] They noted a marked increase in deaths from myocardial infarction among the no treatment group (5% versus 0% in patients treated with estrogen). Unfortunately, details regarding preexisting disease are incomplete, making the subsequent difference in cardiovascular disease between the two groups more difficult to interpret.

More recently data have been collected on patients who have undergone surgical staging. ERT after surgical Stage I and II endometrial carcinoma was found to be associated with a decrease in overall recurrence rate.[13] Although the numbers of patients in each subgroup are small the recurrence rates remain lower when stratified for grade and stage. There was no significant difference in disease-free survival between the two groups. There was, however, an increase in intercurrent disease in the non-HRT group.

The major limitation to all of the existing data is the retrospective nature of the studies, leading to numerous biases, especially selection bias. However, it can certainly be concluded that there is no dramatic increase in the recurrence rate among patients who are treated with HRT following endometrial carcinoma. The currently available data suggest a possible improvement in the disease-free interval for estrogen treated patients. While it appears that there may also be an improvement in overall survival due to a decrease in intercurrent disease, this difference may also be due to inherent selection bias as was seen in the most recent study.

In 1997, the National Cancer Institute (NCI) with the Gynecologic Oncology Group began a prospective randomized double-blind trial of ERT versus placebo in women with a diagnosis of surgical Stage I or II endometrial adenocarcinoma. Therapy started within 12 weeks of surgical treatment. This study is expected to accrue over 2,000 participants, and will provide a definitive answer to the important question of ERT in women with a history of endometrial carcinoma. It is interesting to note that while the addition of progestins has been shown to be beneficial in women with intact uteri who are using ERT, there are no data to show a similar benefit in women with a personal history of endometrial cancer. The ongoing prospective study will only address the use of unopposed estrogen. Until these results are available, the American College of Obstetricians and Gynecologists Committee

Opinion has concluded that women with a history of endometrial carcinoma may be considered for ERT using the same criteria applied to other women. However, prognostic factors should also be taken into consideration.[14] Of course all women considering ERT should be counseled regarding the potential risks and benefits.

BREAST CANCER SURVIVORS AND MENOPAUSE

Breast cancer is the most common cancer among women. Nearly 180,000 women were diagnosed with breast cancer in 1998 and over 43,000 will die of the disease.[1] However, the number of women surviving breast cancer continues to increase. Of the 8.25 million Americans estimated to be alive with cancer in 1998, nearly a quarter of them, over 2 million, are women with breast cancer (Figure 13.1). The 15-year survival rate overall for all women diagnosed with breast cancer is 60%. For women diagnosed with early-stage disease under the age of 75, the 15-year survival rates are over 80%, and for women diagnosed with regional disease, 10-year survival rates in all age groups are over 50%.[15]

Most women with breast cancer are postmenopausal when diagnosed, and the majority of women who are diagnosed when premenopausal are at risk of premature menopause as a result of systemic adjuvant chemotherapy. Although the risk is related to the type of drug therapy administered and increases with age, the overall risk of amenorrhea is approximately 70%, and is nearly universal in women older than age 45.[17]

Postmenopausal breast cancer survivors experience not only the usual symptoms of estrogen withdrawal (i.e. hot flushes, dyspareunia, urinary tract infections, sleep disturbances and mood changes) but also are at risk of mortality associated with cardiovascular disease and osteoporosis.[18] Moreover, women who experience premature menopause are at increased risk of coronary heart disease, a risk which is reduced by ERT.[19]

Women who survive breast cancer not only experience the usual symptoms of menopause, but also live long enough to be at risk of cardiovascular disease and osteoporosis. Estrogen replacement therapy (ERT) or hormone (estrogen plus progestin) replacement therapy (HRT) offer both the promise of improved quality of life, and protection from the

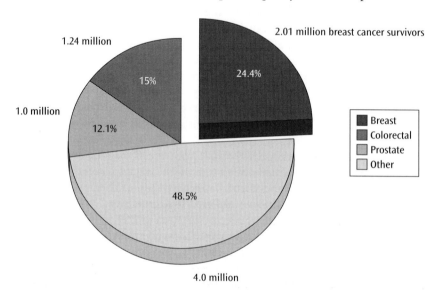

Figure 13.1 *Estimated number of Americans living with cancer in 1998.*[16]

morbidity and mortality associated with cardiovascular disease and osteoporosis. Unfortunately, the standard of care today proscribes using ERT or HRT for breast cancer survivors. Alternatives to hormone therapy which offer both symptomatic relief and reduced cardiovascular and osteoporotic risk in breast cancer survivors have yet to be proven in clinical trial. It is essential, therefore, not only to understand the relative risks and benefits which ERT/HRT may offer breast cancer survivors, but also to be aware of new strategies which will ameliorate the symptoms and mortality risk associated with menopause, yet not increase the risk of either recurrent or new breast neoplasms.

THE ROLE OF ESTROGEN IN THE CARCINOGENESIS OF BREAST CANCER

Breast cancer risk factors

Major risk factors for developing breast cancer include age, family history, certain types of benign histological findings on breast biopsy, and reproductive history. Contributing risk factors include also radiation, lack of physical activity and obesity, dietary fat intake, and alcohol use. Early menarche, late menopause, nulliparity, age at first live birth all increase the risk of developing breast cancer and reflect measures of the cumulative effects of estrogen and progesterone on the developing and mature female breast.[20] A model of breast cancer carcinogenesis is represented best as a complex, multi-stage sequence of events (Figure 13.2). Interactions among genetic, environmental, dietary, hormonal, and other yet to be understood events, occur over years and result in the alteration of normal breast epithelium. What follows is the promotion of biological processes which cause cellular proliferation, the emergence of cellular atypia and non-invasive neoplasia, and ultimately, invasive malignancy capable of metastasis.[21] Estrogen (whether endogenous, or

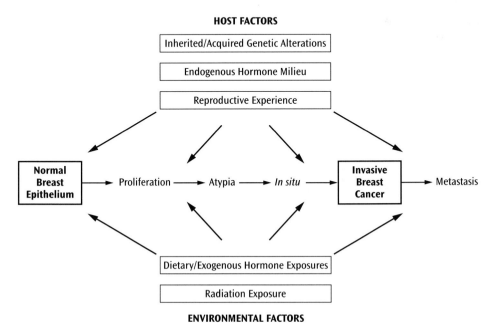

Figure 13.2 *The interaction of environmental and host factors in a multistage model of breast carcinogenesis.*

exogenous) is not the primary carcinogen in this model, but rather acts as a promoting agent at multiple sites in a cascade of events which ultimately results in the development of breast cancer. The promoting effects of estrogen are proposed to include interactions with genetic susceptibility factors such as abnormal genes known to be associated with breast cancer (*BRCA 1*, *BRCA 2*, *p53*), metabolic perturbations of estradiol metabolism, alcohol consumption, and interactions with estrogen receptor expression on normal breast epithelium.[22,23]

Breast cancer risk and exogenous hormone therapy

Women are exposed to exogenous estrogens through the use of oral contraceptives and ERT/HRT. Oral contraceptives have been in use throughout the world for over 30 years. Although the relationship between oral contraceptive use and the risk of breast cancer may be controversial, there appears to be no protective effect observed.[20] Of concern, however, is the evidence from population-based case and cohort studies which suggests an increased risk of developing breast cancer among women who reported more than 10 years of use before age 45.[20]

Evidence from meta-analyses[24] and from long-term prospective follow-up studies consistently demonstrate decreased overall mortality among postmenopausal women receiving HRT. However, the overall mortality benefit appears to be attenuated because of the increased risk of breast cancer associated with long-term HRT.[25] An increased risk of developing breast cancer among women with prolonged use (>5 yrs) has been a consistent finding in studies of ERT/HRT.[20] In an early meta-analysis the risk of breast cancer increased significantly for each year of estrogen use.[26] In the prospective Nurses Health Study cohort the risk of breast cancer was significantly increased among women who were current users of either ERT alone, or HRT compared with post-menopausal women who have never taken hormones.[27] An additional increase in the risk of breast cancer was associated with more than five years' use of ERT/HRT, and the addition of progestin did not reduce the increased risk of breast cancer among the postmenopausal women studied. Additional studies support the conclusion that short-term ERT/HRT (<5 yrs) has no important effect on the risk of breast cancer, and that the addition of progestin neither increases nor decreases the risk of breast cancer further.[27,28] Although women with a positive family history of breast cancer may be at additional risk of developing breast cancer when they use ERT/HRT, they nevertheless also enjoy an overall decrease in mortality compared with women who have never used ERT/HRT.[25,29]

These studies suggest the overall conclusion that while prolonged ERT/HRT in post-menopausal women may be associated with an increased risk of breast cancer, use of ERT/HRT for up to five years is clearly associated with overall decreased mortality from cardiovascular and osteoporotic events, and is not associated with an increased risk of breast cancer, even among women with positive family history of breast cancer, when compared to women who have never taken ERT/HRT.

If this conclusion is correct, ERT/HRT may have a role in reducing overall mortality among postmenopausal women with a history of breast cancer by having a relatively greater effect on the reduction of mortality from cardiovascular and osteoporotic events than it does on increasing the relative risk of breast cancer mortality.

HORMONE REPLACEMENT THERAPY IN WOMEN WITH A HISTORY OF BREAST CANCER

Concerns about the potential risk of estrogen therapy in women with a personal history of breast cancer have been expressed for many years. In an early opinion Spicer and colleagues[30] expressed the two fundamental concerns:

1 estrogen has a significant role in promoting the growth of breast cancer
2 individuals with a personal history of breast cancer have a significantly increased risk of developing a second breast cancer

Because of these two concerns, the standard of care which has emerged proscribes the use of ERT or HRT in women with a prior diagnosis of breast cancer, for fear that the primary cancer will be stimulated to recur, and/or the woman will be at increased risk of developing a second breast neoplasm. In an excellent review of the rationale for considering a clinical trial to address the question of ERT in breast cancer survivors, Cobleigh[18] argued that without a clinical trial both clinicians and patients would continue to make decisions without useful data. It was becoming increasingly clear that there was an expanding need to examine both the quality of life and longevity of women surviving with breast cancer. Cobleigh has called for the NCI to support a pilot study to evaluate the feasibility of undertaking a clinical trial to test the benefits of ERT in women with a history of breast cancer. Recognizing the difficulties inherent in undertaking a scientific study of the question, Cobleigh addressed methodological issues such as concerns that the estrogen effect on breast parenchyma would alter the sensitivity of follow-up mammograms, that for women taking Tamoxifen there existed the potential for both beneficial and harmful drug interactions, and that women might or might not even be willing to participate in such a trial. Additional calls for an organized clinical trial to examine the question have been raised[31–33] based on uncontrolled obersvations that suggest ERT would not be harmful to women with a prior history of breast cancer.[34–36] One large study, in particular, even suggests a protective effect of continuous progestin.[37]

Prompted by an NCI workshop on 'Clinical Trials of Hormone Replacement Therapy in Patients with a History of Breast Cancer', Perlman and Ford studied longevity projections of the effects of Tamoxifen plus progestin versus HRT in breast cancer survivors.[38] Under even the most optimistic assumptions HRT was projected to provide no longevity benefit; under the worst case parameters, HRT was associated with a decrease in expected survival exceeding −2.0 years, while Tamoxifen plus progestin was associated with an increase in expected survival of +0.5 years. The projections varied little by stage, risk of heart disease, or hysterectomy status. Based on these models the NCI concluded that there would be no rationale to study HRT in breast cancer survivors and therefore has no plans to undertake symptom relief or disease prevention studies in breast cancer survivors. Tamoxifen plus progestin studies are currently under way.

ALTERNATIVES TO ESTROGEN/HORMONE REPLACEMENT THERAPY IN BREAST CANCER SURVIVORS

In a recent review Colditz[39] argued for caution and informed consent in recommending ERT in breast cancer survivors. Although short-term ERT/HRT may be unlikely substantially to increase the risk of breast cancer recurrence in women with a history of breast cancer, the uncertainty of the risk in an individual woman demands that alternatives to estrogen-based treatments should be actively explored.

A number of alternatives to ERT to manage menopausal symptoms and postmenopausal cardiovascular and osteoporotic risks have been reviewed.[40] Vasomotor symptoms may be managed by nonestrogen hormonal therapy (primarily progestins), non-hormonal agents such as clonidine or Bellergal, and nonpharmacological interventions such as dietary and behavioral modifications of triggers for hot flushes. Vaginal symptoms may be ameliorated by moisturizers, lubricants, and regular sexual activity; vaginal estrogen preparations with low systemic absorption are also available. Nonestrogen treatment approaches for post-menopausal osteoporosis include exercise, vitamin D and calcium supplementation, bisphosphanate therapy, and newer, selective estrogen receptor drugs.[40,41] Reduction in risk of cardiovascular disease is associated with healthy lifestyle factors which include dietary modifications, exercise, control of obesity, and smoking cessation. Good control of hypertension and diabetes also contribute to reduced risk of cardiovascular mortality. An increasing number of women are exploring complementary and alternative therapies which include behavioral and massage therapy, herbal and homeopathic remedies, and acu-puncture.[40] A complete review of these strategies is beyond the scope of this chapter. However, newer pharmacological approaches which selectively target estrogen receptor activity differently in different target tissues, promise new opportunities to provide 'ideal' postmenopausal symptoms and disease risk management.

New pharmacologic approaches

The 'ideal' agent for pharmacological intervention in the postmenopausal woman might be described as attentuating the vasomotor symptoms associated with menopause, selectively exerting an anti-estrogen effect on the breast and uterus, maintaining bone density, altering cholesterol and lipid profiles favorably, maintaining urogenital epithelial integrity, and being noncarcinogenic.[42,43] In breast cancer survivors Tamoxifen has been the mainstay of postmenopausal anti-estrogen therapy. Tamoxifen provides major benefits in women with established breast cancer by both reducing the risk of recurrence by approximately 30% in the adjuvant treatment of the primary neoplasm, as well as reducing the risk of developing a second cancer in the opposite breast by nearly 50%.[44,45] However, despite the observation that Tamoxifen retards the loss of bone density,[46] produces a favorable effect on lipid and lipoprotein levels,[47] and may be associated with decreased cardiovascular mor-tality,[48] it is associated also with vasomotor and vaginal symptoms, as well as the risks of fatal thromboembolic events and endometrial cancer.[49] Tamoxifen has recently been demonstrated to reduce the expected incidence of breast cancer among high-risk women by nearly 50%, reproducing the decreased incidence of second breast cancers observed in patients being treated with Tamoxifen for primary breast cancer.[50] The positive results of the Breast Cancer Prevention Trial are tempered by the risks of fatal thromboembolic events and the increased risk of uterine cancer, and re-emphasize the need to develop more selective estrogen receptor modulators for women at high risk of developing breast cancer, as well as for women with established breast cancer who require treatment to ameliorate postmenopausal symptoms and to decrease the risk of cardiovascular and osteoporotic events.

New anti-estrogens are being developed which may have a more favorable profile of activity than Tamoxifen in postmenopausal women (Table 13.1). Toremifene (chlorota-moxifen) is approved for use as an anti-estrogen in metastatic breast cancer. Although toremifene does not appear to produce liver tumors in rats, the drug is less potent than

Table 13.1 *Agonist (+)/antagonist (−) effects on selected target tissues by selected anti-estrogens compared to estrogen*

	Breast	Uterus	Bone	Lipids	Vasomotor stability	Liver carcinogen
Estrogen	+	+	+	+	+	+
Tamoxifen	−	+	+	+	−	+
Toremifene	−	+	+	+	−	−
Raloxifene	−	−	+	+	−	−

Tamoxifen and remains associated with vasomotor symptoms as well as a mild estrogenic effect on the uterus.[42] Raloxifene, recently approved for the treatment of osteoporosis, results in a decrease in bone resorption and lowers low-density lipoprotein cholesterol concentrations. It has no demonstrable estrogenic effect on the uterus although long-term data are not yet available.[41,51] Raloxifene prevents the development of mammary tumors in animal models. Initial results of the MORE trial of raloxifene in postmenopausal women showed a decrease in risk of breast cancer as well as a possible decrease in the risk of endometrial cancer with approximately two years of follow-up.[52] These findings, if confirmed in follow-up trials, would have important implications for all postmenopausal women.

SUMMARY

The number of cancer survivors in the U.S. continues to increase. Women with a personal history of breast or endometrial cancer remain at risk of menopausal symptoms, as well as the morbidity and mortality associated with cardiovascular and osteoporotic events. Whereas HRT has become standard for menopausal women without a history of breast cancer, the increased risk of breast cancer associated with prolonged estrogen use makes it relatively contraindicated for women with a personal history of breast cancer. Tamoxifen has been established to be of benefit in women with a history of breast cancer, and more recently as a breast cancer prevention strategy for women with increased risk of developing breast cancer. Its agonist/antagonist profile with vasomotor and urogenital symptoms, and increased risk of endometrial cancer and thromboembolic events results in Tamoxifen being less than ideal as the hormonal therapy of choice for postmenopausal breast cancer survivors. For the present, short-term (>5 years) ERT/HRT may be offered to selected, fully informed breast cancer survivors who are at low risk of recurrence of their disease, and who require relief of unacceptable and unmanageable postmenopausal symptoms, or are at increased risk of significant cardiovascular or osteoporotic events. To date ERT/HRT has not been shown to be significantly disadvantageous for postmenopausal women at increased risk of developing breast cancer.

For survivors of endometrial cancer, participation in the ongoing prospective trial of ERT must be a priority in order to obtain a definitive answer for the survivors of the future. The limited retrospective data that are available support the use of estrogen therapy in selected patients with early-stage endometrial cancer who have undergone appropriate counseling regarding potential risks and benefits.

New drugs with more selective estrogen receptor agonist/antagonist activities may prove to be appropriate for the millions of women who are breast cancer survivors and the millions more who are at increased risk of developing breast cancer during their lifetime. As these drugs are developed and their clinical profiles are defined they may prove to offer important advantages over ERT/HRT for these women.

REFERENCES

1 Landis SH, Murray T, Bolden S, Wingo PA: Cancer Statistics, 1998, *CA Cancer J Clin*, 48: 6–29, 1998.

2 Barakat RR, Park RC, Grigsby PW, Muss HD, Norris HJ: Corpus: Epithelial tumors. In: Hoskins WJ, Perez CA, Young RC, eds. *Principles and Practice of Gynecologic Oncology*. Philadelphia, PA: Lippincott-Raven, 1997.

3 Grady D, Gebretsadik T, Kerlikowskek, Ernester V, Pettiti D: Hormone replacement therapy and endometrial cancer risk: a meta-analysis. *Obstet Gynecol* 85: 304–313, 1995.

4 Nyholm HCJ, Nielsen AL, Norup P: Endometrial cancer in postmenopausal women with and without previous estrogen replacement treatment: comparison of clinical and histopathological characteristics. *Gynecol Oncol* 49: 229–235, 1993.

5 Laferty F, Helmuth D: Post-menopausal estrogen replacement: the prevention of osteoporosis and systemic effects. *Maturitas* 7: 147–159, 1985.

6 Pettiti DB, Perlman JA, Sidney S.: Non-contraceptive estrogens and mortality: long-term follow-up of women in the Walnut Creek Study. *Obstet Gynecol* 70: 289–293, 1987.

7 Ettinger B, Golditch IM, Friedman G: Gynecologic consequences of long-term unopposed estrogen replacement therapy. *Maturitas* 10: 271–282, 1988.

8 Paganini-Hill A, Ross R, Henderson B: Endometrial cancer and patterns of use of estrogen replacement therapy: a cohort study. *Br J Cancer* 59: 445–447, 1989.

9 Pike MC, Peters RK, Cozen W, Probst-Hensch NM, Felix JC, Wan PC, Mack TM: Estrogen-progestin replacement therapy and endometrial cancer. *J Natl Cancer Inst* 89: 1110–1116, 1997.

10 Premarin Package Insert. Wyeth-Ayerst Laboratories.

11 Creasman WT, Henderson D, Hinshaw W, Clarke-Pearson DL: Estrogen replacement therapy in the patient treated for endometrial cancer. *Obstet Gynecol* 67(3): 326–330, 1986.

12 Lee RB, Burke TW, Park RC: Estrogen replacement therapy following treatment for Stage I endometrial carcinoma. *Gynecol Oncol* 36: 189–191, 1990.

13 Chapman JA, DiSaia PJ, Osann K, Roth PD, Gillotte DL, Berman ML: Estrogen replacement in surgical Stage I and II endometrial cancer survivors. *Am J Obstet Gynecol* 175(3): 1195–1200, 1996.

14 ACOG Committee Opinion. *Estrogen Replacement Therapy and Endometrial Cancer*. August 1993; Number 126.

15 Wingo PA, Gloeckler Ries LA, Parker SL, Heath, Jr CW: Long-term cancer patient survival in the United States. *Cancer Epidemiology, Biomarkers & Prevention* 7: 272–282, 1998.

16 Stat Bite. Persons living with major cancers in the United States, 1998. *J Natl Cancer Inst* 90: 565, 1998.

17 Osborne CK, Clark GM, Ravdin PM: Adjuvant systemic therapy of primary breast cancer. In: Harris JR, Lippman ME, Morrow M, Hellman S, eds. *Diseases of the Breast*. Philadelphia, PA: Lippincott-Raven, 548–578, 1996.

18 Cobleigh MA, Berris RF, Bush T, *et al*: Estrogen replacement therapy in breast cancer survivors. *JAMA* 272: 540–545, 1994.

19 Stampfer MJ, Colditz GA, Willett WC, *et al*.: Postmenopausal estrogen therapy and cardiovascular disease. Ten-year follow-up from the Nurses' Health Study. *N Engl J Med* 325: 756–762, 1991.

20 Henderson BE, Bernstein L: Endogenous and exogenous hormonal factors. In: Harris JR, Lippman ME, Morrow M, Hellman S, eds. *Diseases of the Breast*. Philadelphia, PA: Lippincott-Raven 185–200, 1996.

21 Helzlsouer KJ: Early detection and prevention of breast cancer. In: Greenwald P, Kramer BS, Weed DL, eds. *Cancer Prevention and Control*, New York, NY: Marcel Dekker, INC: 509–535, 1995.

22 Zumoff B: Does postmenopausal estrogen administration increase the risk of breast cancer? Contributions of animal, biochemical, and clinical investigative studies to a resolution of the controversy. *P.S.E.B.M.* 217: 31–37, 1998.

23 Khan SA, Rogers MA, Khurana KK, Meguid MM, Numann PJ: Estrogen receptor expression in benign breast epithelium and breast cancer risk. *J Natl Cancer Inst* 89: 37–42, 1997.

24 Grady D, Rubin SM, Petitti DB, *et al.*: Hormone therapy to prevent disease and prolong life in postmenopausal women. *Ann Intern Med* 117: 1016–1037, 1992.

25 Grodstein F, Stampfer MJ, Colditz GA, *et al.*: Postmenopausal hormone therapy and mortality. *N Engl J Med* 336: 1769–1775, 1997.

26 Steinberg KK, Thacker SB, Smith SJ, *et al.*: A meta-analysis of the effect of estrogen replacement therapy on the risk of breast cancer. *JAMA* 265: 1985–1990, 1991.

27 Colditz GA, Hankinson SE, Hunter DJ, *et al.*: The use of estrogens and progestines and the risk of breast cancer in postmenopausal women. *N Engl J Med* 332: 1589–1593, 1995.

28 Stanford JL, Weiss NS, Voigt LF, *et al.*: Combined estrogen and progestin hormone replacement therapy in relation to risk of breast cancer in middle-aged women. *JAMA* 274: 137–142, 1995.

29 Sellers TA, Mink PJ, Cerhan JR, *et al.*: The role of hormone replacement therapy in the risk for breast cancer and total mortality in women with a family history of breast cancer. *Ann Intern Med* 127: 973–980, 1997.

30 Spicer D, Pike MC, Henderson BE: The question of estrogen replacement therapy in patients with a prior diagnosis of breast cancer. *Oncology* 4: 49–59, 1990.

31 Eden JA, Wren BG: Hormone replacement therapy after breast cancer: a review. *Cancer Treatment Reviews* 22: 335–343, 1996.

32 DiSaia PJ, Grosen EA, Kurosaki T, Gildea M, Cowan B, Anton-Culver, H: Hormone replacement therapy in breast cancer survivors: a cohort study. *Am J Obstet Gynecol* 174: 1494–1498, 1996.

33 Sands R, Studd J: Hormone replacement therapy for women after breast carcinoma. *Current Opinion in Obstetrics and Gynecology* 8: 216–220, 1996.

34 Peters GN, Jones SE: Estrogen replacement therapy in breast cancer patients: a time for change? *Proc Annu Meet Am Soc Clin Oncol* 15: A148, 1996.

35 Bluming AZ, Wile AG, Schain W, *et al.*: Hormone replacement therapy (HRT) in women with previously treated primary breast cancer. *Proc Annu Meet Am Soc Clin Oncol* 15: A203, 1996.

36 Vassilopoulou-Sellin R, Theriault R, Klein MJ: Estrogen replacement therapy in women with prior diagnosis and treatment for breast cancer. *Gynecologic Oncology* 65: 89–93, 1997.

37 Eden JA, Bush T, Nand S, Wren BG: A case-control study of combined continuous estrogen-progestin replacement therapy among women with a personal history of breast cancer. *Menopause* 2: 67–72, 1995.

38 Perlman JA, Parnes HL, Ford LG.: Projections of the longevity effects of Tamoxifen (TAM) + progestin (T + P) versus hormone replacement therapy (HRT) in breast cancer survivors requiring hormonal symptom relief. *Proc Annu Meet Am Soc Clin Oncol* 16: A462, 1997.

39 Colditz GA: Estrogen replacement therapy for breast cancer patients. *Oncology* 11: 1491–1494, 1997.

40 Kessel B: Alternatives to estrogen for menopausal women. *P.S.E.B.M.* 217: 38–44, 1998.

41 Eastell R: Treatment of postmenopausal osteoporosis. *N Engl J Med* 338: 736–746, 1998.

42 Gradishar WJ, Jordan VC: Clinical potential of new anti estrogens. *J Clin Oncol* 15: 840–852, 1997.

43 Jordan VC: Tamoxifen; the herald of a new era of preventive therapeutics. *J Natl Cancer Inst* 89: 747–749, 1997.

44 Early Breast Cancer Trialists' Collaborative Group: Systemic treatment of early breast cancer by hormonal, cytotoxic, or immune therapy: 133 randomized trials involving 31000 recurrences and 24000 deaths among 75000 women. *Lancet* 339: 71–85, 1992.

45 Early Breast Cancer Trialists' Collaborative Group: Tamoxifen for early breast cancer: an overview of the randomized trials. *Lancet* 351: 1451–1467, 1998.

46 Love RR, Mazess RB, Barden HS, *et al*.: Effects of Tamoxifen on bone mineral density in postmenopausal women with breast cancer. *N Engl J Med* 326: 852–856, 1992.

47 Love RR, Wiebe DA, Newcomb PA, *et al*.: Effects of Tamoxifen on cardiovascular risk factors in postmenopausal women. *Ann Intern Med* 115: 860–864, 1991.

48 Costantino JP, Kuller LH, Ives DG, Fisher B, Dignam J: Coronary heart disease mortality and adjuvant Tamoxifen therapy. *J Natl Cancer Inst* 89: 776–782, 1997.

49 Fisher B, Dignam J. Bryant J, *et al*.: Five versus more than five years of Tamoxifen therapy for breast cancer patients with negative lymph nodes and estrogen receptor-positive tumors. *J Natl Cancer Inst* 88: 1529–1542, 1996.

50 Wickerman DL, Costantino JC, Fisher B, *et al*.: The initial results from the NSABP Protocol P-1: a clinical trial to determine the worth of Tamoxifen for preventing breast cancer in women at increased risk. *Proc Annu Meet Am Soc Clin Oncol* 17: A3A, 1998.

51 Bryant HU, Dere WH: Selective estrogen receptor modulators: an alternative to hormone replacement therapy. *P.S.E.B.M.* 217: 45–52, 1998.

52 Cummings SR, Norton L, Eckert S, *et al*.: Raloxifene reduces the risk of breast cancer and may decrease the risk of endometrial cancer in postmenopausal women. Two year findings from the multiple outcomes of raloxifene evaluation (MORE) trial. *Proc Annu Meet Am Soc Clin Oncol* 17: A3, 1998.

Index

Note: page numbers in *italics* refer to tables, those in **bold** refer to figures.